The 40-Day *Body Image* Workbook

*Hope for Christian Women
Who've Tried Everything*

Heather Creekmore

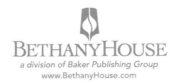

BETHANYHOUSE
a division of Baker Publishing Group
www.BethanyHouse.com

Published by Bethany House Publishers
Minneapolis, Minnesota
www.bethanyhouse.com

Bethany House Publishers is a division of
Baker Publishing Group, Grand Rapids, Michigan

Printed in the United States of America

Library of Congress Cataloging-in-Publication Data
Names: Creekmore, Heather, 1974– author.
Title: The 40-day body image workbook : hope for Christian women who've tried everything / Heather Creekmore.
Other titles: Forty-day body image workbook
Description: Minneapolis, Minnesota : Bethany House Publishers, a division of Baker Publishing Group, [2023]
Identifiers: LCCN 2023026947 | ISBN 9780764241956 (paperback) | ISBN 9781493443864 (ebook)
Subjects: LCSH: Christian women—Religious life. | Body image in women—Religious aspects—Christianity. | Spiritual exercises.
Classification: LCC BV4527 .C776 2023 | DDC 248.8/43—dc23/eng/20230717
LC record available at https://lccn.loc.gov/2023026947

Cover design by Micah Kandros Design

Published in association with Books & Such Literary Management, www.booksandsuch.com.

Baker Publishing Group publications use paper produced from sustainable forestry practices and post-consumer waste whenever possible.

23 24 25 26 27 28 29   7 6 5 4 3 2 1

To every woman who's ever
ordered a salad when she really craved a burger;
watched an infomercial, made the payments, and hoped for a miracle;
bought an overpriced bottle of product that made her hair worse; or
believed that pounds, inches, or skin elasticity defined her worth.

You are seen, you are valuable, and you are loved.

This book is for you.

Contents

To the One Who's Tried Everything

I have no idea how I ended up with type B blood because every ounce of my personality is type A. Give me a plan; I'll work it. Give me a goal; I'll try to reach it. This is the book I never wanted to need. Certainly, with enough effort, an overachiever like me could find her way out of body image issues.

But no amount of planning or striving ever led me to a place where the scale and mirror sang, "You are so beautiful." One look at my thighs, and the only thing I heard was the *Mission: Impossible* theme.

Maybe you feel the same right now. Perhaps frustration furrows through your mind. It doesn't seem fair that you're still trying to make peace with your body after all you've done. Why won't God just zap this all away? Why does *this* have to make the to-do list?

If you're like me, maybe you had a grand plan to shrink your body image issues into oblivion. As soon as you found the "right" diet or exercise program that fit your life, you'd watch your concerns magically disappear.

Or perhaps you thought you'd age out of your body image issues. Did you believe that by the time you were twenty, thirty, forty, fifty, or older, you'd feel so settled in your skin that you could blow those body image issues away like the flickering candles on your cake? *I sure did.*

I see you if you've logged hundreds of prayers asking God to take this away from you. I know you if you looked at the before-and-afters, bought the plan, and felt hopeless when the results didn't follow. I hear you when you say that you've literally "tried everything" but nothing seems to make a difference. You still don't like the way you look.

I've been there.

Of course, decades ago, I would have told you my problem was with my body, not my body image. I was sure that all the negative feelings about my appearance would resolve if I just changed how I looked. Obsessive thoughts would cease. My disordered relationship with food and exercise would vanish. As soon as I found the right formula to fix it all, my body image would transform.

But the ducks never lined up, at least not in a way that freed me spiritually, physically, mentally, and emotionally from my body image struggle. Instead, those thoughts of my inadequacies quacked daily, hourly, and sometimes every minute. They plagued me even when I finally wore the size I'd always hoped to wear.

God has done a makeover on my heart. Though my teen daughter is the only one who can fit into my old sizes, today I'm free in a way I never thought I could be. It's been almost a decade since I wrote my first book, *Compared to Who?*, which chronicles how God led me out of body image bondage. That book, my blog, and my podcast have offered me the opportunity to coach other women who, like me, have fought a nonstop battle with the number on the scale or their reflection in the mirror.

Many of my clients had read other body image books. They knew that God and *Vogue* have different definitions of beauty, but they were still stuck. Why couldn't they just break free? Working with each woman for six weeks, I gave them homework: reading and journaling assignments. The work wasn't always easy, but over time, they felt a sense of freedom they'd never before experienced.

Freedom. That sounds nice, doesn't it? Can you imagine what life would be like if you didn't have to obsess over every calorie? What if the words "Let's take a picture!" no longer made you want to go hide in the bathroom? How would it feel to confidently wear shorts in the summer or a swimsuit at the beach? What would it be like to see your reflection in the mirror and not spiral into negative thoughts?

Maybe you doubt this kind of freedom is actually possible. Perhaps you've ridden up the escalator of hope so many times, you can't bear the thought of another letdown. Through the pages that follow, I offer encouragement so that

- you can know and feel like you are loved beyond what you measure.
- you can be free from the judgment of the scale and the dressing room mirrors.
- you can experience the freedom of entering a room without fearing what others think of your body.

And trust me, friend: When this change happens on the inside, you radiate a type of beauty that Photoshop and touch-up filters can't match.

Diets and body "makeover" plans promise that we'll get their results if we follow their rules. But body image freedom isn't about getting the rules right. The freedom to accept, appreciate, and make peace with your body doesn't come from a perfectly executed plan. It comes from determining to walk a new path.

One client of mine, Amanda, has been on this path for over a year now. We followed a course similar to the one laid out in this book as we worked together. Today, she texted me this:

> I can't even count how many times I've said to my husband, "I'm so happy now." I'm seriously a different person. Even my twelve-year-old commented on how different and relaxed I've been lately—and she doesn't even know what I've been working to change. I knew I was struggling. I knew I was obsessed and consumed. But I didn't know how much bondage I was in until I got free.

I invite you to read and work through these biblical concepts I've used with hundreds of coaching clients. There are questions to help you process, exercises to apply what you're learning, and Scripture verses to help you hear God's heart in your struggle and to keep you close to the only one who can truly help you change. You may choose to slow down as you work through the content. Some concepts may trigger thoughts that will take a few days or more to process. You may want to read through the entire book first and then go back to the beginning and do the exercises. There's no time pressure. Just keep working on it regularly, and you will make progress.

You'll find questions strategically placed throughout each chapter, but you'll also find special "Work It Out" and "Act" sections. "Work It Out" is designed to help you actively process what you've read, while "Act" offers bonus activities for those ready to take the content and concepts to the next level of application.

Many books are dedicated to making sure you feel good about yourself. But feeling good about yourself is a temporary condition that's subject to change—sometimes hourly. The type of transformative journey in this book is designed to last. That's why we go deep. Afterwards, you may even feel empowered to invite other women out of their bondage and into freedom with you.

We have so much more to offer the world than our ability to shrink or transform our bodies. God created us on purpose and for a purpose. I know that's hard to believe in our image-focused culture.

Today, I invite you on a journey to see your body image issues in a completely new way. Healing your body image is vital to your physical, mental, and spiritual health. We'll explore how to reset your programming about food and your appearance, and why you care so much about them both. Will you join me?

Start by taking the following quiz. Then, when you're finished with the book, read and sign the Certificate of Commitment on page 221 to treat yourself with grace as you walk a new path to body image freedom. I can't wait to see how God begins to set you free.

Body Image Quiz

1. On an average day, I think about the way I look . . .
   a. Multiple times a day.
   b. What is an average day? Some days I plan out my next diet all day long, but other days I don't worry about it.
   c. Occasionally. But seeing that woman on a billboard or on TV really does make me think about my flaws. . . .
   d. Rarely. I'm a wash-and-go girl. I don't know what I weigh or what my hair looks like right now.

2. When I think about my body, my first thought is . . .
   a. Gross. I hope no one ever has to see this unclothed with the lights on.
   b. If I could just change this, and this, and this, then I would smile in the mirror.
   c. Some days I'm gorgeous. Some days I'm not.
   d. I can't wait for swimsuit season.
   e. I am who I am. This body is temporary.

3. The last time I went on a diet or an "eating plan" was . . .
   a. Monday. In fact, I'm on one right now.
   b. I try new eating plans whenever I hear about them, but I wouldn't call it "dieting."
   c. Can't remember, but I've tried many over the years.
   d. I eat what I want to eat and don't stress over food.
   e. What is a diet?

4. If I were completely honest, I'd have to say that I exercise because . . .
   a. I want to change something about my body.
   b. I have to burn up some calories.
   c. I want to look better.
   d. It's a great stress-reliever.
   e. Define *exercise*. I move my body because it makes me feel good.

5. When I hear, "It's what's on the inside that counts," I think . . .
   a. That's nice, but it doesn't apply to me.
   b. Whatever. That may be true, but I still need to look good on the outside too.
   c. I know deep down this is true. But I still have a hard time believing it (or acting like it's true) most days.
   d. Encouraged. Yes. God loves me. Every time I hear it, I feel freed from thinking about my body.

6. This is how much time I spend thinking about food each day . . .
   a. All. Day. Long.
   b. I carefully calculate my macros and/or calories.
   c. Some days I'm consumed. Some days I don't remember what I ate for lunch.
   d. I forget to eat sometimes.
   e. I have no clue. Do people really think about food? That's a thing?

7. When I think about swimsuit season, I think . . .
   a. Ugh. Why does summer come every year? Can I wear yoga pants to a pool party? I loathe swimwear.
   b. Okay, it's three months away, so I will workout every day and eat salads for dinner, and I'll be ready.
   c. I'm ready, I just need to find a good tummy-controlling swimsuit.
   d. Woo hoo! Who's hosting the pool party?
   e. I don't really give it too much thought.

8. Have you ever had this thought: *If I could just lose (or gain) ____ pounds, then I would be happy?*
   a. Hourly.
   b. Daily.
   c. Only when I'm trying on clothes.
   d. My weight isn't something I think about.

9. I'd really like for other people to see me as physically beautiful.
   a. True. This is important to me.
   b. True. I wish this wasn't important, but it is.
   c. True sometimes, but only when I put in the effort to look nice.
   d. False. Who cares? It's what's on the inside that counts.

10. If other people compliment my appearance, I feel . . .
    a. Indifferent. They're just being nice (or lying).
    b. Anxious. If people don't say anything about my appearance, I wonder if I look bad.
    c. Good. It helps to know that other people think I look good.
    d. I don't really care what others think of my appearance.
    e. Great! I say "Thank you!" and smile for the rest of the day.

11. How do you feel when you see images of so-called "perfect" women?
    a. Imperfect.
    b. They make me feel like I'm not enough.
    c. I try to remind myself that they're airbrushed, but I still wish I looked more like that.
    d. It doesn't faze me. It's what's on the inside that counts, right?
    e. Indifferent. We are all unique.

12. Bad hair days, pimples, bloating, or the number on the scale will affect my day in this way:
    a. I'll feel lousy all day. Confidence gone.
    b. Another day I have to be devoted to finding new skincare, a new hairdresser, or a new diet.
    c. I'll do occasional mirror check-ins on my flaws, but the day isn't ruined.
    d. Why let a little issue like that ruin a perfectly good day?

13. Inside my head, I hear . . .
    a. Constant criticism and judgment: *You are too fat, too ugly. Why did you eat that?*
    b. Lies: *No one loves you. They think you're ugly. You have no value.*

  c. A mixture of thoughts. Some days I fight lies, criticism, and judgment. Other days I feel confident.

  d. I'm not sure.

  e. Affirmation: *I am made in God's image. I am loved.*

14. I've thought this: *If I could just be more like her, then I would be happy* . . .

  a. Hourly. It would feel great to have a body that's more like hers.

  b. Daily. Every time I look in a mirror.

  c. Sometimes, but I try to push that thought down and remind myself of the truth.

  d. I've never thought that.

15. I really wish there was a way for me to stop worrying about what I look like and stop obsessing over my appearance.

  a. True. And I know that this will happen when I lose weight and get my body the way I want it.

  b. True. And I wonder if there is some spiritual root of this issue I just haven't figured out yet.

  c. True, but I'm trying to work on a more positive mindset regarding my body image and mental health.

  d. True and false. It depends on what day you catch me!

  e. False. I don't really spend time stressing about this.

Scoring:

Count and write down the totals of each answer below.

A: _____

B: _____

C: _____

D: _____

E: _____

For every answer of A or B: give yourself 5 points

For every answer of C: give yourself 3 points

For every answer of D or E: give yourself 1 point

My Score: _____

50 points or more: Body Image Is a Beast

You're battling the body image beast! Some days it feels like you are in the fight for your life as you try not to be consumed by the pressures to lose weight or change your appearance. You may be battling a full-blown eating disorder, or you may just have an anthem of negative thoughts and lies about your appearance and worth charging through your head most of the day. The enemy lies to you a lot. He tells you that you aren't worthy or you need to look different in order to be worthy of love. You need help battling these lies and uncovering why they keep you stuck. You worry that your negative feelings about your body will never change. For best results, tell someone that you're working through this book, and ask them to keep you accountable. Hopelessness and despair are two of the enemy's best tricks to keep us from making progress. Include a friend or family member who can encourage you to keep working at it. Don't be afraid to seek additional help from a Christian counselor or therapist as you work through thoughts or memories that are difficult or painful.

30–49 points: Body Image Is a Bother

You aren't overly obsessed with changing the way you look, but every once in a while, body image bogs you down. Like an annoying mosquito, the enemy whispers in your ear that you need to change. You get hung up on trying to eliminate cellulite, change the number on the scale, erase the wrinkles, or flatten those abs. Body image feels like a roller-coaster ride. Some days you cruise without care, and other days you feel like screaming. You long to find consistency and reach a place where you can feel at peace with your body. This workbook should offer great support for your journey and help you uncover why certain triggers impact your body image more than others.

29 points or fewer: You Keep Body Image Issues at Bay

You're doing a great job making peace with your body and not stressing much over your body image. But body image issues can build over time. Use this book as a guide to help you continue to work through those body image flare-ups that may trigger behaviors or thought patterns that could lead to a bigger struggle with body image issues in the future.

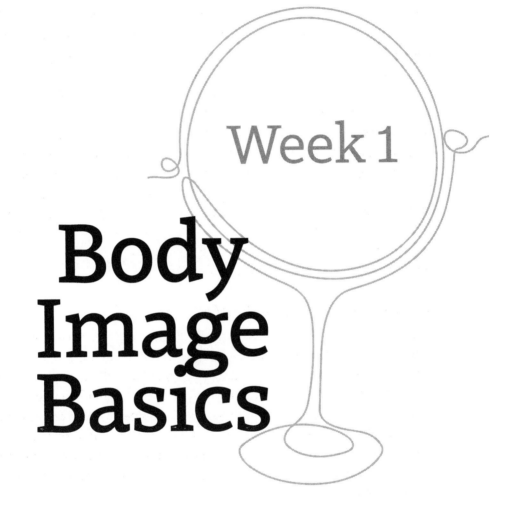

Week 1

Body Image Basics

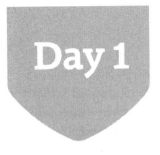

You're Like Abraham

Get ready for a journey to a foreign land of body acceptance

> Your heart, mind, hands, and feet are stamped with the imprint of the Creator. Little wonder that the Devil wants you to be ashamed of your body.
>
> *Joni Eareckson Tada*

I bet you didn't expect a body image book to start by comparing you to one of the patriarchs of the Old Testament. Granted, there aren't an abundance of similarities. But trust me, friend. Your journey to body image freedom and Abraham's adventure to a new land may be more similar than you think.

In Genesis 12, the Lord tells one of the most famous men in the Bible to leave everything familiar. He promises to bless Abraham and bring blessing to future generations if Abraham will follow the Lord's lead out of Haran. Notice that God doesn't tell him an exact address to pop into his phone's navigation system. Instead, he calls him to "the land I will show you" (v. 1).

For most of us, the journey to seeing our bodies biblically is a venture into unknown territory. You look at the woods and wonder if there's really a trail through those trees.

The land I will show you? Yikes! I would've asked God for more information before loading my bags on the camel. I like to know where I'm going, when I'm going, and how I'll get there. Oh, and I'll pack snacks and a bottle of water. *I never leave home without a full water bottle.*

Yet, implicit in God's command to Abraham is a call to trust. Verse 4 tells us, "So Abram went, as the LORD had told him." Perhaps we're supposed to learn from his quick obedience. **Can we trust God to lead us to a place—mentally, physically, and spiritually—where we are at peace with our bodies?**

Changing the Programming

I said the sinner's prayer before I could tie my shoes. I've been following Jesus for most of my life. Christian schools, a Christian college, even a Christian graduate school characterized my education. I knew the gospel and all about Jesus's sacrifice for me. But trusting God hasn't always been easy—especially in the arena of my body. **I could surrender my heart but not my dress size.**

Now I work with women who face a similar battle with their body image. They're tired of stressing over food and letting the scale dictate their mood. They want to be free, but their brains are on autopilot. They don't know how to think about or see their bodies in any other way.

And I get it. You can't just flip a switch and fix your body image issues overnight. These patterns of thinking and believing weren't developed in a day, so they'll take some time to change. But change is possible. I know it is. I've experienced it.

A Foreign Land

Whether you've been battling your body image for a week or a lifetime, the days ahead may feel like a journey to a foreign land. Seeing our bodies through the lens of the gospel stands antithetical to almost everything in our culture. A woman who isn't always trying to lose weight, obsessed with her size, fretting over body parts, wrinkles, or hair? That woman is going to stand out from the crowd.

She's an enigma.

She's countercultural.

She may not get thousands of Instagram likes.

I confess. I've been on a decade-long quest to try to be more like that kind of woman. It's still a challenge some days. Stand with any group of women around a dessert table, and you'll only have to wait a few minutes before someone comments about the calories in the cookies. Go out to dinner with a group of gals, and I can almost promise someone will use the words "I'm being good" in the context of the food they order. Diet culture language combined with the over-emphasis on physical appearance has turned many of us into food apologists. We empathetically nod along when someone quips, "Those go straight to my hips" or "I'll go to the gym and work it off later."

If you're like me, this is a familiar land where you Google the trendiest diets and workouts so you can speak the dialect with ease. If Whitney from work is cutting carbs, you try it too. **We all chase the same dream, sharing our tips and tricks along the way. In our culture, this is how women relate to one another.**

I barely passed economics—it was a video course, and the instructor was dreadfully dull. Alas, the economy of our native land is straightforward: Weight loss = praise. Success stories revolve around someone ruthlessly shedding pounds to get "healthy." A high value is placed on your ability to appear as if you have it all together. Look good, and you'll get good. Look better, and there's no limit to the joy life will bring. *Sigh. So much pressure!*

A Different Way

This feels a little different from how God's kingdom works. Okay, maybe a lot different. God doesn't define success, beauty, or health the same way we do. Likewise, any journey toward having a more biblical view of body image may feel like boarding a spaceship to Mars. When you're the only one *not* on a new diet, *not* making negative comments about your body, or *not* uber-focused on what you're wearing, you feel like an alien.

Isn't that a bundle of encouragement?

Oh, friend! Freedom is worth it. I know the joy, peace, and rest found in trusting God and choosing the alternate path. **Obsessing over our bodies has made us anxious, stressed, and depressed. There's another way!**

It's not always easy. Culture touts body transformation as the gateway to all joy. Like dog hair on your black pants, brushing culture's claims fully off is practically impossible. Yet, like Abraham, it's time to enter a new land, turn in a new direction, and leave the old behind. Chances are you've tried the plans. You've bought the diet foods, crunched your way through eight-minute abs, or read copious articles on losing weight for life. This is an invitation to try a new way—to approach your body image struggles as matters of the heart, not the body.

The best news is this: You're not alone on this journey. God is for you. No matter what you've walked through—be it a full-blown eating disorder; frustration with your height, your skin, or your hair; or decades of yo-yo diets—you've not disappointed God. His grace will cover you as you walk through this wilderness. Will you accept his invitation to journey to a new view of you?

Work It Out

Write about your body image journey so far. Are there areas where you've been stuck for a long time? Use any of the applicable prompts below to help.

Here's what I've wished I could change about my body . . .

No one knows this about my body image struggle . . .

Read Genesis 12:1–3 and Galatians 5:1. Has your body image struggle become so familiar that not having it would feel foreign?

Galatians 5:1 talks about the "yoke of slavery." Has body change ever felt like bondage to you? How so?

What would body image freedom mean for you?

My Goals

Are there specific habits or patterns in your life that you would like to break through on this journey? Here are some examples:

· I'd like to feel okay wearing shorts in the summer.
· I want to stop yo-yo dieting.
· I'd like to feel confident enough to not have to change clothes multiple times before leaving the house.

Goal 1: _____

_____

_____

Goal 2: _____

_____

_____

Day 2

You're Like Sarah

It takes faith to believe God can fix this

> Now to him who is able to do far more abundantly than all that we ask or think, according to the power at work within us . . .
>
> *Ephesians 3:20 ESV*

Now that you've established some goals for your journey, let's look at how the path ahead may differ from others you've traveled.

You see, I tried just about anything to change my body. I'm the reason infomercials work. When it comes to a supplement that will zap me skinny, my faith is fierce. Sure, there's cynicism too. I argue, *Won't this fail like all the others?* But my faith wins. If there's even a slight chance this could be the miracle that solves all my food and body issues, why risk missing out?

I've spent countless dollars on exercise gizmos, downloadable food plans, and make-me-slender supplements. Sometimes my confidence helps them work for a week or two. (*Likely the placebo effect.*) I swallow the first pill and instantly feel my stomach shrink. But imaginary results eventually wane. I give up. Defeated. Once again, my purchase let me down. Has this ever happened to you?

The book of Hebrews lauds Abraham as a man of great faith in God. Like we talked about yesterday, he picked up and left his homeland without so much as the name of his destination.

But Abraham's faith wasn't perfect. Yes, he exudes trust as he sets out on the journey to a mysterious promised land, but let's pick up the story a little later when his faith was challenged. God made Abraham a promise—he'd be the father of many. Yet Sarah, his wife, was infertile. At seventy-six years old, she gave up and told old Abe to sleep with her maid, Hagar.

Let me repeat that. *She gave up at seventy-six!*

Hagar has a son for Abraham, but the Lord tells Abe that Ishmael isn't the one he's been waiting for. After a heavenly visit where God's promise was repeated, Sarah becomes pregnant and births a baby boy. As a reminder of Sarah's response to how preposterously amazing this act of God was, the couple named the baby Isaac, meaning laughter. In Genesis 21:6, Sarah says that "everyone who hears about this will laugh with me." In Genesis 21:1, the Bible tells us that the Lord was "gracious" to Sarah, and he did what he promised. His grace poured out on her, even though she had trouble believing.

So, back to your body image. How's your faith? **Do you believe that God can** *actually* **change this area of your life?** I ask the women I coach what their number one hesitancy is about working together. The most common response is, "I'm afraid it won't work. Nothing else has!" *Maybe you even had that thought when you bought this book!*

Tried All the Things

Perhaps like me, you've tried all the things. Some worked for a season; some never worked. You've tried fitness plans and diets. You've tried surgeries or undergarments that make it look like you've had surgery. Powders, pills, creams, injections, and supplements. *Check.* You've looked in the mirror and told yourself you're pretty. You've dutifully written lists of what you "appreciate" about your body. Yet the Ferris wheel never lets us off the ride. Our heads won't stop spinning. **We hope a few body tweaks will settle our worth and stop the cycle altogether. But deep down, we all wonder,** *Will I ever be free?*

Can you relate? List any aspects of your struggle that you feel will never change:

On a scale of 1 to 10, how important of a goal has body improvement become in your life?

1 ········ 2 ········ 3 ········ 4 ········ 5 ········ 6 ········ 7 ········ 8 ········ 9 ······ 10

Not important   Somewhat important   Very important

On a scale of 1 to 10, how confident are you that God can heal your body image issues?

1 ········ 2 ········ 3 ········ 4 ········ 5 ········ 6 ········ 7 ········ 8 ········ 9 ······ 10

Not confident   Somewhat confident   Very confident

Fighting Disappointment

Our body image journey can feel like one long string of letdowns. We're disappointed that the plan didn't work (or the results didn't last). Maybe we're frustrated with how much we've been working out or spending on skincare products, yet we still don't like the way we look. The struggle could be with aging. None of the turn-back-the-clock potions rewind time well enough.

Maybe it's deeper than that. Maybe you just feel depressed that this is the body God gave you, and you wrestle a twinge of resentment. How is it fair that "this" is the body he chose for you?

Circle the types of disappointment that resonate the most with you today:

I'm disappointed by fitness/nutrition plans that didn't work.

I'm frustrated I've wasted money on plans that didn't work.

I'm disappointed that results from previous plans/efforts didn't last.

I'm frustrated I've wasted time and my body image still isn't better.

I'm disappointed that this is the body God chose for me.

I'm frustrated that God didn't make me look different.

I'm disappointed that I can't stop the effects of aging.

Where Have We Placed Our Faith?

I can relate to every one of the feelings on the list. But let's go back to square one. There's only one kind of hope that does not disappoint. As Romans 5:5 reminds us, that's the hope placed in the one who could never disappoint: Jesus. When I put my faith in counting points or riding a fancy exercise bike, it's misplaced hope. These body transformation tools may change my physical being, but they won't touch the places where my body image needs the most healing—in my heart and in my mind.

*Read Genesis 18:14 and Genesis 21:1. Genesis 18:14 asks, "Is anything too hard for the L*ORD*?" How does Sarah's story inspire you to believe that God can do a miracle in this area of your life?*

Work It Out

Write a letter to God about the disappointment you've felt over your body.

    Dear God,

_____

_____

_____

_____

_____

_____

_____

Day 3

You're Valuable

Understanding the economics of worth

> Your worth is not determined by the opinions of God's other creations.
>
> *Heather Creekmore*

A few decades ago, I was worth about twenty camels. Yes, I mean the tall desert animals with the humps. Despite inflation, I'm not sure if I'd be worth that many now. *Aging is real.*

I was on a trip to Israel for a class. It was my first real out-of-the-country experience (aside from that hour I spent in Tijuana just to say I'd been to Mexico). After visiting a holy shrine, we crossed paths with an Arab man. One of my classmates, Dan, engaged him in cordial conversation, but soon I heard our new Arab friend say, "I'll give you twenty camels for the blond girl."

Dan laughed and said it was a tempting offer, but he didn't think he could get the camels in his carry-on. *Thanks, Dan.*

Later we asked a local to explain. Trading camels for a young woman was a standard transaction. At the time, a camel was worth two to three thousand U.S. dollars. That meant my value to this man settled somewhere in the ballpark of $50,000.

Wearing a price tag feels odd and uncomfortable. It conjures disturbing and disgusting images of slave trade and trafficking. To put a monetary value on any human life is to miss the heart of God. Our value is immeasurable. But I wonder if this same immeasurability is what makes it so difficult for us to comprehend our value.

Worth Seven Years' Wages

Remember Sarah and Abraham? Their son, Isaac, found a wife of his own, and the couple welcomed twin boys: Jacob and Esau. There's interesting family drama here, but eventually Jacob grows up and leaves home to find a wife. He quickly falls lovestruck for a girl named Rachel. So enamored, he offers to work for her father for seven full years to pay for her. *I guess that's not too different from the camel arrangement.*

Jacob was like a preschooler with a new iPad. Seven years went by, and Scripture tells us it felt just like a day to him. With his debt worked off, it was finally time for him to receive his prize—the beautiful Rachel. But then something downright tragic happens. Laban, Rachel's father, decides to do a little bait and switch. Instead of giving Rachel to Jacob at the wedding, Laban subs in her older (and less attractive) sister, Leah. Leah and Jacob spend the night together, and it's only the next morning when Jacob realizes he's been duped.

We'll explore more of this story later, but I feel heartsick for poor Leah. I wonder what she felt like she was worth. Rachel, her younger sister, was worth seven years' wages, but Dad didn't think he'd get anything for Leah, so he threw Leah at Jacob like the bonus donut that comes in the baker's dozen.

Am I Valuable?

At some level, we all question our value. Sadly, part of me felt affirmed by the camel proposition. My boyfriend moved across the country, then decided that long-distance relationships weren't for him. Combine that with my body image issues, and I felt unwanted. The offer of $50,000 made me feel a pinprick of worthiness. Still, I secretly wondered if the offer would have been higher if I were prettier.

If the question of your value has ever echoed through your heart, then let's take a fresh look at where our worth comes from. **The very premise that we were created in God's image has been undermined by culture for decades. Is this why we struggle to believe we're valuable?**

No Creator, No Value

When my son was in kindergarten, he brought home little books that wove this message into each story: "Remember when that big explosion created the world . . ." Each time we read it, we tried to re-teach him. "No, Zach, this isn't true. God made the universe, and each of us too." As parents, we knew our assignment was bigger than getting him through his homework.

While what children learn about the universe's origin may seem trivial to your body image issues, stay with me here. The confusion over our creation has a more significant impact than we see. According to the "Millennials in America" study, Dr. George Barna explains the damaging impact of a whole generation that never learned they were created on purpose. It's easy to feel like an off-brand bargain when you don't know you were divinely designed.

Barna believes that seeing ourselves as happy accidents tremendously impacts the mental health crisis this generation faces. He explains the harm that can come from not believing in the presence of an omnipotent and loving Creator:

> Without any anchors for truth, emotions, decision-making, relational boundaries, or purpose, a sense of anomie and disconnectedness is only natural.[1]

What connections do you see between understanding how God created us and knowing our worth?

Did you grow up learning that you were intrinsically valuable because God created you? If so, jot down some of the lessons you learned and who shared them. Or, can you remember if or when you heard this message in adulthood?

How does this truth make you feel?

---

1. George Barna, "Millennials in America: New Insights into the Generation of Growing Influence," Foundations of Freedom, October 2021, https://www.arizonachristian.edu/wp-content/uploads/2021/10/George -Barna-Millennial-Report-2021-FINAL-Web.pdf.

The Economics of Value

It only takes a few minutes of scrolling Instagram to figure out what culture values. Success stories revolve around the person who can accomplish the biggest transformation in their body shape, bank account, or number of followers. Wisdom, integrity, and faithfulness are no longer tradable commodities. Beauty, wealth, and celebrity are the Park Place and Boardwalk on our culture's Monopoly board.

We've become so untethered from the foundations of where our true worth is derived that we flounder. Our souls can't know their worth apart from Jesus. **You can wear the size, have the look and the flawless skin—but until you know you're valuable inside, you'll never feel valuable on the outside.**

In the Christmas carol "O Holy Night," there's one line that always strikes me: "He appeared and the soul felt its worth." Jesus completes the puzzle. He's the answer to every economic problem our hearts face. Only he can fill that hole in our soul.

What are you worth? You're worth what someone is willing to pay for you. And I have tremendous news. Jesus paid it all.

Work It Out

Have you ever struggled to believe you were valuable or "worthy"? Write about it here.

What have you observed from culture's lessons about what makes a person valuable?

If God were to respond directly to the messages you hear about not having value or worth, what do you think he would say?

Read Genesis 29:15–30. How did you feel as you read Jacob and Rachel's love story? What attributes beyond physical beauty do you ascribe to Rachel? What attributes do you ascribe to Leah?

Read Leah's response in Genesis 29:35. After you've completed this workbook, what would have to happen for you to be able to say, "This time I will praise the LORD"?

How would it feel to experience this kind of contentment in life and in your body image?

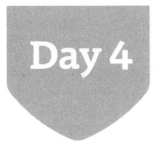

Day 4

You're Not a Project

Paint-your-own-pottery theology

> You are not a problem to be solved.
>
> *Geneen Roth*

I didn't think the whole way through my purchase of the Total Gym. Thirty minutes into watching Chuck Norris talk about its wonderful features, I knew if it was good enough for a super ninja, it was good enough for me! In four to seven business days, I'd tone like a champion.

There were only a few miscalculations in my plan. After missing the delivery window twice, UPS kindly decided to keep my package at the distribution center. I ventured to their hidden warehouse to proudly exchange my claim card for my body-makeover-in-a-box. *It can't be that heavy.*

Oh, but it was.

I managed to get the monstrous box in my vehicle and then home, where I pushed it out of my SUV and onto my garage floor. The box and I danced up one little step into the kitchen and then held a mini pep rally before tackling the main stairs.

Soon I was reminded that what slides up can also slide down. In case you're wondering, a ninety-pound box can gain enough momentum sliding downstairs to nearly flatten a woman. It took me a solid thirty minutes, with several breaks to give myself motivational speeches—"You got this, Heather"—before I got that Total Gym up all sixteen stairs.

The Total Gym and I were BFFs for two whole weeks. Until one day when I had to fold it into the corner so some guests would have room to sleep. Apparently, Chuck and I do not have the same definition of "stores easily." The Total Gym never came out again.

Sigh. I'm a marketer's dream. If there's a slim chance a product could be as awesome as promised, why not try it? Getting the Total Gym set up almost sent me to the hospital, but I'm not complaining. *Those twelve workouts were totally worth it.*

I'm kidding. But understand there's nothing comical about the job of a marketer. They must ensure that you know you are not enough. That may sound severe, but follow me. **There's a much better chance of you buying their product if they can find the area in your life where you are discontent and offer you a solution to fix it.**

When we feel like we lack, we do more, buy more, and strive more. But this discontent also plays a supporting role in our body image issues. We believe the subtext of the beauty marketers' messages. We see our bodies as a blank slate designed for improvement.

But you are not a first draft waiting for edits. You're not a fixer-upper hoping HGTV stars will renovate you to greatness. Our biggest purpose isn't to get a rounder bottom or sculpted abs. **When we view our bodies as projects, we view ourselves as objects.**

In what ways have you viewed your body as a project?

Paint-Your-Own Pottery

Scripture's reference to jars of clay in the book of 2 Corinthians reminds me of the many visits I've made to those paint-your-own-pottery places. I'm fabulously awful at it. My creations are so bad that I always "forget" to retrieve them after they've gone in the kiln.

I had a paint-your-own-pottery view of my body. I believed God had given me a blank vase—a jar of clay—and it was my job to make it the prettiest jar around. Sure, God molded and formed the creation, but my job was to take his work and make it look good.

This responsibility for beautification felt like it was part of my divine purpose. Even the church seemed to reinforce this message. "Be a good steward of your body" certainly sounded like I should reshape, mold, paint, and prettify what God created.

"Well done my good and faithful servant" would surely come after reaching my goal weight and toning my arms. Then, like a doting father, God would be proud of me, as if getting a better body was an amazing achievement for his kingdom.

But my perspective was skewed. **Now I see that healing our body image issues is more about correcting our theology than correcting our biology.** Scripture mentions little about what we do with the outside of our vessels. Second Corinthians 4:7 reads like this, "But we have this treasure in jars of clay, *to show that the surpassing power belongs to God and not to us*" (ESV, emphasis mine).

Now, don't get me wrong, the jars-of-clay part is significant. We're all a little unique, just as no two pieces of pottery are exactly alike. Jars of clay were also referred to as earthenware. This is such a fascinating word, given that our bodies are what our souls "wear" while we're on earth.

But this treasure inside that Paul refers to is the light of the gospel. It's the illumination of "the knowledge of the glory of God in the face of Jesus" (2 Corinthians 4:6 ESV). We are containers for his light and his grace. Our beauty comes from his radiance. If we want to emit beauty, we don't have to change our bodies, we just have to let that radiance out!

There's Nothing Wrong with Your Vessel

Compared to the true beauty of the One who fills us, even the "best" physical body is still frail and common, weak, weathered, and filled with imperfections. If you feel like a first draft, a less than, or a have-not in a world of beautiful bodies, can I encourage you? **There's nothing wrong with your vessel.**

Though the marketers won't stop mocking, and you may fall prey and dance with a Total Gym or two, understand that God has given you everything you need physically to accomplish his purpose for your life. As the Westminster Catechism reminds us, the chief end of man is to know God and make him known. **Your body is fully equipped for this mission, no matter your age or build, skin condition, or size.**

I love how Mother Teresa put it: "I'm a little pencil in the hand of a writing God, who is sending a love letter to the world." You don't have to change your body to be used by him.

Work It Out

Have you ever felt like you were a first draft that someone was waiting for you to improve?

In what ways have you watched others pursue body improvement?

Did their success or failure in this arena impact how you viewed them?

Did their success or failure give them more value?

Read 2 Corinthians 4. Do you ever struggle to believe the true treasure is inside of you?

How does this chapter help you to believe the truth about your value?

Act

Pay attention to your thoughts about your body and start a log.

We become so familiar with these ongoing, recurring thoughts that often we no longer notice what they're saying. **The first step in breaking free from the shaming voices in your head is to stop and listen.**

Start the log in a notebook you carry with you or in the Notes app on your phone. Record any negative thoughts or lies and what triggered them. *It will be hard to hear them at first.* But keep this log going for a few weeks until you can clearly identify the shaming thoughts you have most often.

Here's a framework for you to use of examples of thoughts and what may have caused them:

Date	Thought	Precipitating Event
Monday, January 2	*I'm so fat. I have to lose weight.*	*Getting on the scale. Feeling like my jeans got tighter.*
Wednesday, January 4	*No one will ever love me with skin like this. I look gross.*	*Scrolling Instagram. Seeing photos of friends/women with flawless skin.*
Friday, January 13	*I am lazy. I'll never change.*	*Watching weight loss commercial.*

You're Not Recyclable

Understanding God's design of our bodies

> For we know that if the earthly tent we live in is destroyed, we have a building from God, an eternal house in heaven, not built by human hands.
>
> *2 Corinthians 5:1*

I never wanted to look like Barbie—consciously, at least. I knew her feet were too small and her legs too slim to support her height and a bust that size. Plus, my cousin decided my dolls were the perfect place to practice her haircutting skills. Most of my Barbies looked like they'd been styled with a Weedwacker. *Apparently, I grew up with body image issues for both myself and my Barbie dolls.*

But there's something alluring about the concept of body perfection. Whether it's the airbrushed image on a slick magazine cover or an iconic doll who drives a pink convertible and lives in a dream house, life in plastic does seem fantastic. Isn't *flawless* the goal those cosmetics companies tell us to shoot for? Yet, I wonder. **The more we strive to look like plastic dolls, the further it seems we get from God's design for our bodies to image him.**

You see, polymers—the molecules of plastic—were invented. You and I, on the other hand, were created. But how many of our body goals sound like we're trying to be more plastic?

We "firm up" so we can be "rock hard." We strive to eliminate anything jiggly or squishable. We smooth and tone to help skin look flawless. When you think about those terms—*firm, hard, smooth*—it sounds a lot like I'm describing plastic.

But check the bottom of your feet. I'm pretty sure there's no number 5 stamped inside a small triangle of arrows designating your appropriate bin. **You, my friend, are not recyclable.**

And when you compare your body to, let's say, a red Solo Cup, there are many obvious distinctions. The human body is a living organism. It's always changing. It can look and feel different every day. It appears more supple in its youth than it does in maturity. It responds naturally to the climate, the weather (*Hello, humidity! My hair feels you!*), and our activities. A photo of your face during the week before your period might look different than a photo of it the week after.

For example, your stomach miraculously expands (up to five times its original volume[1]) to accommodate a large meal until your intestines have time to digest it all. By morning, sometimes it will have shrunk again. Other times it's still working to digest the number of tortilla chips you consumed.

And every day, you have a choice. You can try to eat less or consume only the foods that can be digested quickly so, like those plastic dolls, your stomach never changes size. Or you can respond to your body's God-given hunger signals and eat until full without fretting over natural stomach expansion. You can live free from the bondage of overthinking the process of digestion. You can view your body as an amazing living organism equipped and capable of turning Mexican food into usable energy. You may even fill with awe as you consider how many elaborate processes happen inside your body each day.

Friend, we're not inanimate objects. Our bodies change. We have parts that don't look or function like anything a machine could ever mass-produce.

You Were Formed

That's how God designed us. Shaped. Formed. Scripture uses each of these words to describe our bodies. **Though I love watching the ocean or gazing at the stars, we are the most magnificent of all of God's creations.**

One trip to the zoo, and you can see God's love for diversity. Animals weren't made in the image of God—yet they display his fantastic creativity. Can you imagine if every animal looked like a tiger? These cats are striking creatures,

---

1. Maged Rizk, "Does My Stomach Actually Shrink When I Lose Weight?" Health Essentials, August 18, 2020, https://health.clevelandclinic.org/does-my-stomach-actually-shrink-when-i-lose-weight/.

yet how blah would the zoo be without monkeys, pink flamingos, giraffes, or black-and-white zebras?

Think of an animal you like. What characteristics of this animal make it your favorite?

In what ways can you see how God created this animal with certain characteristics on purpose and for a purpose?

Original Design

God created us fearfully and wonderfully. More than 70 trillion possible combinations of traits are determined by your DNA.[2] This is more than the total number of people who've ever lived! You're undoubtedly an original.

Conversely, plastic comes from a mold. Formed pieces that look different from the model get tossed off the assembly line. Imperfection renders them unusable. **But our variety is an asset.** It's how we tell each other apart! With so many different possible combinations of features, shapes, and sizes, it's impossible to define "perfection" in the realm of our human bodies. In fact, it's hard to replicate someone else's look without intervention. Makes you rethink the term *plastic surgery*, right?

Please hear no guilt, shame, or condemnation if you've had work done. If you've undergone a nip, tuck, or augmentation just for the fun of it, God isn't mad at you. I've worn colored contacts, push-up bras, and Spanx. The only difference is the price and the permanence.

Instead, I want to encourage you. Surgeries don't solve body image issues. I have women reach out to me every month who've gone for the procedure they were confident would fix their body image issues, only to be left with a giant bill and more uncertainty.

2. Dennis O'Neil, "Biological Basis of Heredity: Recombination and Linkage," 2013, Palomar College, https://www.palomar.edu/anthro/biobasis/bio_3.htm.

We're created humans with original designs, not molded plastics. I hope this truth will help encourage and reframe how you think about your body today. It's okay to have a changing body, because that's what human bodies do.

Work It Out

In what ways have you subconsciously treated yourself as plastic or believed your body should be more plastic?

When is it most difficult to believe your body is acceptable, beautiful, or worthy of love?

Read the creation story in Genesis 1, focusing on verses 20–31. What do you observe about God's intentionality in creation? Does God seem content with his creation?

Act

~~~~~~

Today you will write a new motto.

The goal is to replace the theme running through your brain from "It's never enough" or "Keep improving" to something like "God has already given me, physically, everything I need to accomplish his purpose for my life." Or "God knew what he was doing when he made my body." Or "God created me on purpose, for a purpose."

Choose a phrase that resonates best with you, or write your own below. You could even choose a favorite Bible verse if you prefer.

Print and post it somewhere you will see it or can access it quickly—on your mirror, your computer, or even your phone lock screen. Your goal is to begin to replace those condemning thoughts with this new motto.

My Motto

_____

_____

_____

_____

_____

Day 6

You're Staying Positive

Why body positivity isn't enough to be free

> As water reflects the face, so one's life reflects the heart.
>
> *Proverbs 27:19*

I was a busy college student with a thousand things to think about that were *far* more important than watching the gas gauge. But when I pressed the pedal and my Oldsmobile started bucking, I sensed trouble.

Fortunately, we'd just passed a gas station. Twenty minutes later, red gas can in hand, my friend Heidi and I headed back to the stalled car. *Easy peasy!*

I popped open the tank and refreshed that thirsty sedan. Then, triumphantly, I strutted to the driver's side to get in. But the door was locked. *Oh no!* Peering into the driver's side window, I spied our only hope of making that vehicle run again.

As I think of how our culture offers to "fix" body image issues, I'm transported back to that day. The tank had enough gas. But without those keys, I had no power to make the car go (or even open the door!).

There are many options out there to fill your body image "tank." One of the most popular is called body positivity. Surely as Christians, feeling positive about our bodies is a logical choice. We know we shouldn't be body *negative*. **But is body positivity the right movement for Christians to align with?**

41

I don't think so. When I think of body positivity, a famous saying from Inigo Montoya's character in *The Princess Bride* comes to mind: "You keep using that word. I do not think it means what you think it means."[1]

Before I break down *body positivity*, let me reaffirm that your body is good because God made it. He created the whole amazing universe, and he created you. **Because you're made in his image (Genesis 1:26-27), you can rest in the truth that your body is valuable, worthy, and useful.** Be positive about that!

Yet, I'm leery of body positivity. I've watched the movement for more than a decade. At first, it seemed like the answer every woman with body image issues longed for. Finally, someone recognized that if the only bodies we saw on screens were skinny and flawless, we'd create a culture where every girl felt bad for not having that type of body. *Hooray for recognizing this danger!*

But what came next concerned me. On Instagram, I watched women awaken to the truth that their bodies are good, and then park there with pride. Instead of embracing their bodies as a reflection of God's grace and love, they shouted songs of self-love. *Savor your own awesomeness and show your middle finger to any who don't see it.*

Feeling empowered by body boldness is like filling the car with gas but being locked out of the cab. You may have the temporary confidence to post beach selfies, but the deeper heart work is left undone. **We can pep ourselves up for a few seconds or seasons, but only confidence that comes from Christ has staying power.** Body pride doesn't free us from our body shame; only Jesus's healing power can do that.

It's important to understand what we're agreeing with when we say we're "body positive." Yes, God made our bodies good. We can be positive about that. But body positivity preaches a different gospel than the Bible. Here are a few of the main differences between the teachings of body positivity and the Bible:

---

1. *The Princess Bride*, directed by Rob Reiner (1987; Twentieth Century Fox).

Body Positivity Versus the Bible

Body Positivity	*the Bible*
"Beauty is not a single image, but the active embodiment and celebration of self."[2]	All beauty is found in and was created by God. (Psalm 27:4; Isaiah 33:17)
Self-love and self-celebration are the goals.	Love God, love others as you already love yourself. More self-love is not the goal of the Christian life. (Matthew 22:36–40; 2 Timothy 3:2)
Look inward to seek freedom from socially designed ideas about beauty.	Seek God to find true beauty and identity in Christ. (1 Peter 3:3–4; 2 Corinthians 5:17; Galatians 2:20)

See through the Semantics

Though subtle, body positivity has offered a giant umbrella for movements that contradict God's design and make self supreme. Yet many Christians have jumped onto the body positivity bandwagon because the semantics sound correct. Words are always first to be co-opted by the enemy. Remember Eve's talk with the serpent back in Genesis? "Did God *really* say, 'You must not eat from any tree in the garden'?" (Genesis 3:1, emphasis mine).

Even mainstream sources agree that body positivity can put too much emphasis on physical appearance. As one awakens to their "true beauty," they begin to fall in love with their appearance. This revival can result in a loss of any other purpose. It reminds me a bit of Narcissus from Greek mythology. He fell so in love with his reflection that he eventually toppled into despair.

Similarly, experts explain that body positivity can lead to other challenges, because the body positive feel pressured to love their bodies more or to always love their bodies.[3]

---

2. From "This is Beauty," The Body Positive, https://thebodypositive.org/thisisbeauty/about/.
3. Kristen Fuller, MD, "Body Positivity vs. Body Neutrality," Verywell Mind, June 30, 2022, https://www.verywellmind.com/body-positivity-vs-body-neutrality-5184565.

How have you observed body positivity in culture?

Have you ever felt pressure to love your body? Or felt frustrated because you couldn't?

Is Positivity the Answer?

Being body positive isn't the same as having a positive body image. Biblically, we're not instructed to love our physical bodies more. We're told to love Jesus and love others as we *already love* ourselves (Matthew 22:37–39). Though some have tried to twist that verse into a biblical justification for body positivity, verse 39 clearly says there are just two commands. There's no secret third command to love your cellulite before you can love the people on your street. The Holy Spirit gives us the resources to love God and others even as we wrestle with our own insecurities and doubts. In fact, the secret to freedom is just the opposite. **When we take our focus off of trying to love ourselves, it's amazing how much more comfortable our bodies feel.**

Read Matthew 22:37–39 and write what you observe:

Positivity Doesn't Last

In June of 2021, pop star Bebe Rexha posted a video of herself dancing in lingerie and asked fans to help her normalize her new body size, shut down body shaming, and embrace self-love.[4]

But seven months later, the singer took to TikTok to share a different message. She's struggling. She gained more weight, and she avoids social media because of it. Rexha told her millions of followers that she's not sure how to help or love herself at this new size.

Pouring positivity on brokenness is like slathering foundation all over a blemish. It may mask, but it can't heal. Body positivity doesn't have the power to actually transform your body image. It offers a shot of adrenaline, but when the buzz wears off, you feel flat. When your body changes, you have to start all over again. Only a gospel-centered understanding and appreciation for the body has the power to set us free for good.

Our goal is to praise God for how he made our bodies and to use them—without unnecessary inhibition—to serve him. If we make our goal body positivity, we focus on the wrong objective. Body image freedom comes when we shift our focus from manufacturing body love to having a greater love for the one who made us and who has a plan for our bodies.

Work It Out

What would it be like to praise God for the body he has given you?

How do you differentiate praising God from body positivity/praising one's body?

---

4. Hannah Southwick, "Bebe Rexha Spreads Body Positivity in Lingerie: 'Normalize 165 Pounds,'" Page Six, June 30, 2021, https://pagesix.com/2021/06/30/bebe-rexha-dances-in-lingerie-for-body-positivity-tiktok/.

Day 7

You're Not Switzerland

The biblical challenges of being body neutral

> The physical part of you is not some piece of property belonging to the spiritual part of you. God owns the whole works.
>
> *1 Corinthians 6:19–20 MSG*

Looking for body confidence? Pop singer Lizzo belts out some ideas rooted in a great manicure, a flauntable hairstyle, and a fiery determination. This hit song has inspired millions to strut their stuff. I'll admit, it's a catchy tune. But I doubt this music-induced body boost lasts too long after the song ends.

Lizzo is no longer a fan of the body-positive movement. She says it's been "co-opted by all bodies" and has become a trend of "celebrating medium and small girls" while bigger people "are still getting the short end of this movement!"[1] Instead, she endorses body neutrality.

Body neutrality focuses on what your body can do rather than what it looks like. It emphasizes how the body functions, and avoids telling people how they should feel about their bodies. Instead of body love, those in the neutrality camp prefer terms like *body acceptance* and *body liberation*. Experts believe that those coming from an eating disorder background may find body neutrality more helpful than body positivity.[2]

1. Megan Stone, "Lizzo Says Body Positivity Movement Has Left 'the Bodies It Was Created For' Behind," ABC News, April 13, 2021, https://abcnews.go.com/GMA/Style/lizzo-body-positivity-movement-left-bodies-created/story?id=77042664.

2. Sara M. Moniuszko, "Lizzo Criticized Body Positivity. Here's What You Need to Know about Body Neutrality," USA Today, April 22, 2021, https://www.usatoday.com/story/life/health-wellness/2021/04/22/lizzo-criticized-body-positivity-what-body-neutrality/7317015002/.

But as Christ followers, we don't get the option to be neutral. God made our physical bodies on purpose and for a purpose. While a religious group called the Gnostics believe that we're souls trapped in evil shells, Christianity teaches something different. C. S. Lewis aptly captures the distinction here:

> Christianity is almost the only one of the great religions which thoroughly approves of the body—which believes that matter is good, that God Himself once took on a human body, that some kind of body is going to be given to us even in Heaven and is going to be an essential part of our happiness, our beauty, and our energy.[3]

Understanding this is fundamental to a healthy body image. If the foundation of what we believe about our bodies isn't constructed from a biblical point of view, then we're building high rises on the San Andreas fault line.

You aren't Switzerland. You don't have to be neutral. You can believe that your body is good.

Your body isn't just a container that once rolled down an assembly line waiting for a machine to squirt in your soul. Scripture tells us that your body was handcrafted. You were knit together in your mother's womb (Psalm 139). You're a special edition.

Do you tend to separate who you are as a person from your physical body?

Look up Psalm 139:13. What do you think of when you picture something being knit together?

---

3. C. S. Lewis, *Mere Christianity* (New York: Harper One, 2001), 98. *Mere Christianity* by C. S. Lewis © copyright 1942, 1943, 1944, 1952 C. S. Lewis Pte Ltd. Extracts used with permission.

Your Body Is a Gift

In elementary school, I handwove a small square pot holder for my mom. It wasn't half as pretty as one she could have bought at Target, but it came from the heart. I chose the colors and intertwined each strip of fabric by hand. I did the best job I could to make that little pot holder a gift that shouted "I love you!"

I realize that as soon as you hear that illustration, you may feel the reality of it. You may think, *Yes, I feel like that sad little homemade pot holder in a world full of beautiful fabrics and silicones.* But please don't miss my point. You weren't tacked together by an elementary school girl who struggled to cut straight lines and thought pink-and-purple was everyone's favorite color combination. No, you were handcrafted by the God of the universe. He didn't rush to finish you before the bell rang. He poured his love into creating you for your good and for his glory.

Can you believe you were handcrafted? What thoughts or images does that truth evoke?

Imagine giving someone a homemade pot holder, and instead of admiring the colors or the pattern, the recipient said, "This is very useful!" Would you feel a little slighted? *I would.* **Most women who struggle with body image issues are much more comfortable feeling useful than they are feeling beautiful.**

We can't be neutral about our bodies because we're not separate from our bodies. I am not me without my body. Genesis shows us that God created Adam's body from the dust first, then breathed life into him and he became a living soul (Genesis 2:7). Adam's body was not an afterthought.

Look up Genesis 2:7. Why do you think God chose to give us bodies?

Are you more comfortable feeling useful than beautiful? Why or why not?

The Body Is Not Nothing or Everything

A theologically sound view of the body is more like this: "Your body is not nothing. Nor is it everything."[4] It's not that the body doesn't matter or is only valuable because of its usefulness. It's that the body only tells one part of the story.

God's outstanding creation does not have to be viewed as utilitarian only. My worth cannot be found in what I do any more than it can be found in what I look like. Both my talents and my thighs were intentionally chosen by God. But my worth can only be found in him.

Know that God didn't mess up when he made you. **Your body is a gift to help you understand who you are and what you were created to do.** Though culture tells us we determine our own destiny and decide who and what we want to be without limits, God has placed us within our bodies, on purpose, with his unique purpose for us.[5]

Body neutrality says, "I love my legs because they help me walk." Body positivity says, "I love my legs because I decide what beautiful legs look like." But a theologically sound view of the body says, "God created my legs on purpose, for a purpose. I can see them as a good gift from him. And because I love him, I'll use them to serve him."

How difficult is it for you to believe that your body was chosen intentionally by God?

Read Ephesians 2:10. What do you observe about how you were created? Can you see connections to your purpose or identify roles or jobs you were not created for?

---

4. Sam Allberry, *What God Has to Say about Our Bodies: How the Gospel Is Good News for Our Physical Selves* (Wheaton, Illinois: Crossway, 2021), 41.
5. Allberry, *What God Has to Say about Our Bodies*, 46.

Work It Out

Think through some of your specific physical attributes. How do these hint at how or what God designed you for?

Act

Your Body Is the Temple

In 1 Kings 6, we read how King Solomon built the temple according to God's instructions. Reading this passage, you can quickly become overwhelmed with the details. God didn't just say, "Build me a temple." He gave specific instructions for size, shape, materials used, and more. In 1 Corinthians 3:16 and 6:19, we read that our bodies are the temple of the Holy Spirit.

Read 1 Kings 6. What do you observe about God's intentionality in building his temple? Can you believe he used the same intentionality when creating you?

Can you believe that the same God who delineated the dimensions of the temple's juniper plank flooring specially made you?

How does it make you feel to know that the same one who determined the exact measurements of the decorative cherubim decided, on purpose, your size and shape?

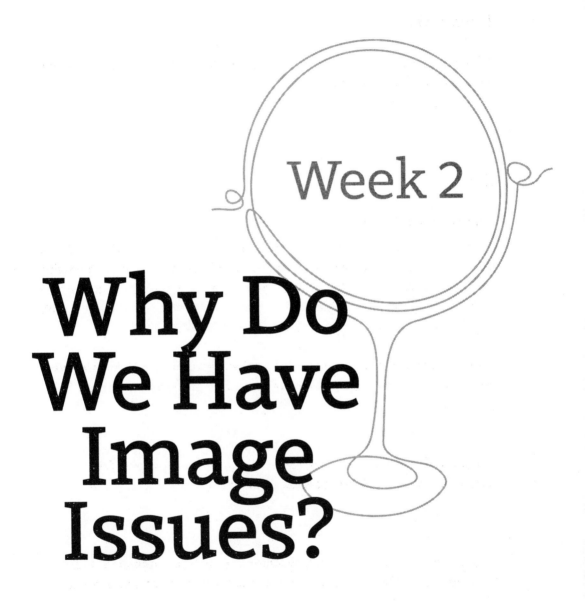

Week 2

Why Do We Have Image Issues?

Day 8

Trusting in the Sweetest Frame

What really keeps us safe

> If you look at the world, you'll be distressed. If you look within, you'll be depressed. If you look at God, you'll be at rest.
>
> *Corrie ten Boom*

I'd never left the house without makeup before. Even a 6 a.m. spin class required some lip gloss and blush. But one day, when I had to skip church (kids were puking, and when your husband is the pastor, there's only one choice of who stays with them!), a friend noticed my absence and stopped by on her way home from service to see if I needed anything.

When she rang the doorbell, my face was bare. It looked like . . . skin! She took one look at me, and she didn't pass out. She didn't shriek with fear or scowl with disgust. Instead, she began a conversation. It was as if nothing was wrong. *It was almost like she didn't even notice.*

I figured she was struggling to hold back the terror she felt inside, so I let her off the hook. I apologized for not having any makeup on. *Yes, that's right.* I told a good friend who knew I'd been up all night with vomiting children that I was *sorry* she had to see my real face. *Maybe you've done this too?*

It's been more than a decade since that encounter, but I'll never forget her response. She said, "Heather, you look about the same."

Wait. What? The same? How could that be? In my mind, this was like saying Cinderella and her ugly stepsisters were tough to tell apart. *Come on!* Maybe she was just being nice.

But a few months later I had the opportunity to participate in a makeup-free experiment. Contributors to a mom blog I wrote for were challenged to post our makeup-free selfies on social media. *Gasp.* You know what I learned? The world didn't stop spinning when people saw me without mascara.

Somewhere hidden inside was this belief that I needed to look a certain way for people to like or accept me. Before marriage, I believed that if I were ever to get a man, it would require me to look the part. But when the ring slid on my finger, that pressure didn't disappear. My image management had been about much more than just finding a guy. How I looked was a vital part of an equation I had constructed for myself. If I look a certain way, then I will be loved. If I don't look a certain way, then no one will even like me.

After reading my story in the previous paragraphs, what resonated most with you? In what ways have you felt pressure or responsibility to make your appearance pleasing to others?

Change Comes When We Feel Secure

Looking back, I see how those who loved me just because of what I looked like didn't last long. I'm not certain if I felt their fakeness and backed away or if they felt my obsession and ran! Either way, relationships that don't go beyond our images are unfulfilling. I guess this is why social media is good for a quick buzz but can cause anxiety and depression long term. Liking one's image does not equate to friendship.

How can I become comfortable without makeup, without wearing the size I want to wear, and without looking the way I want to look? Change comes when we feel secure. Change comes when our identity is placed in something far more trustworthy, admirable, and unchanging than our physical appearance. **And change comes when we know that it's not our body or appearance that will keep us safe—it's Jesus.**

List all the ways your body may change—no matter what you do to try to stop it:

What does this tell you about putting your hope, trust, or faith in body improvement?

Trusting in the Sweetest Frame

There's an old hymn you may have heard called "My Hope is Built on Nothing Less." One line that I've sung for decades recently caught my attention. It goes, "I dare not trust the sweetest frame, but wholly lean on Jesus's name."

Now, I'd guess the author of this song, Edward Mote, wasn't thinking about his body image back in 1834. Yet, I've hoped for a "sweeter frame" to have some security, a place to rest my confidence. If my body looked like I wanted it to, wouldn't it be tempting to put my trust in my own appearance or abilities?

The song, based on the parable of the wise man and foolish man, reminds us that Jesus is the only solid rock where we can build our house—our identity—and be secure. As the Bible story goes, the foolish man built his home on shifting sand. There was nothing solid about that. But when we build on Jesus Christ—the rock, the cornerstone—then we have a rock-solid identity.

Read this parable in Matthew 7:24–27. In what ways is building an identity based on the appearance of our bodies like building a house on the sand?

Think about what it would be like to have your "sweetest" physical frame. What would having that type of body guarantee for you?

No Money-Back Guarantees

Now, look at your answers above. Did you speculate that this better body would guarantee your health? We have no promises that a certain body type will always stay healthy. What about guaranteed approval? Do you believe that having a "better" body will earn you more approval and love? If so, remember that even women with culturally praised body shapes and sizes are rejected, cheated on, and betrayed by friends. *And they still believe they look bad in pictures!*

In reality, we cannot wholly lean on our appearance, our image, or the strength of our bodies to carry us through this life. Sleek bodies wither, and even the strongest bodies break down. There are a few who manage to stay looking youthful until they're eligible for social security, but no one can escape the aging process. This makes our bodies more like the shifting sand than we'd care to admit.

Likewise, beauty doesn't guarantee us security. Think of one of the Bible's most notably beautiful women, Esther. The stunning Esther was plucked from everything and everyone she loved to be part of the king's harem and, after pleasing him in the bedroom, his queen. Then she was asked to use her position of influence and risk her life to save the Jewish people. God blessed Esther with great beauty, on purpose, and for a purpose. But beauty didn't keep her safe; God did. Can we similarly trust that God is the only one who can offer us security?

Work It Out

What will happen if you stay at your current weight, size, shape, or skin condition for the next thirty years?

How will it impact your ability to love your family or others well?

How will it impact God's love for you?

What will happen if you spend the next thirty years stressing over and trying to change your body?

How will it impact your ability to love your family or others well?

How will it impact God's love for you? What could you miss out on?

Is That What I Really Look Like?

Image management 101

> Feeling beautiful has nothing to do with what you look like.
>
> *Emma Watson*

Haven't we all been there? You're laughing, talking, and having a great time. Then someone pulls out their phone and says, "We should take a picture!"

I smile, throw on a little lip gloss, and pray that I don't have to be the person on the end. I make a joke as I fumble to find the most slimming pose. I feel okay about the experience until the photo-taking friend texts the picture to the group. *Oh, please! I hope no one posts that on Instagram!*

Suddenly, the good times stop rolling. The conversation continues, but my mind races through another world. I count every calorie consumed in the past week and begin plotting my body makeover. I obviously need to start a new plan. (Monday, of course.) Then I scheme up ways I could "accidentally" delete the photo from everyone's phone. *Someone needs to invent an app for that.*

I can have a great time and enjoy the company, but when I begin to dwell on what I look like, sound like, or what others think of me, the struggles swirl.

Body Image Isn't Really about Your Body

A decade ago, I was certain my life would be more enjoyable as soon as I improved my body. But body image isn't about our physical forms. Women of all shapes and sizes, ethnicities, and backgrounds can struggle with how they believe they look. Instead, body image is a completely subjective picture or "image" you hold of your own body. Problems ensue when we judge that mental image, determining it isn't as slender or shapely as we'd prefer. We decide the image would be "better" if it were different.

Broadly, image is the picture of ourselves we display to the world. Image can include not only what we look like but how we want others to perceive us. *Do they think I'm kind? Do they see me as successful? What kind of wife/mother/ friend/employee do they believe I am?*

What Kind of Image Do You Try to Portray?

Circle any of these words that apply or add your own:

Successful	Productive	Well-educated	Spiritual
Healthy	Hard-working	Funny	Easy-going
Smart	Energetic	Friendly	In charge
Savvy	Competent	Loving	Attractive
Flawless	Perfect	Talented	Wealthy

Image Management

Enter image management. It's easy to believe that we should (and can) control what other people think of us. Likewise, it's tempting to get caught up in trying to please ourselves with our image. I work with women who struggle in both of these areas. Some worry about what others think when they see them. Some stress over negative thoughts about themselves.

In both cases, image management keeps us primarily focused on perfecting and polishing the outside, while God asks us to submit to him as he cleans and clarifies our hearts.

Read 1 Samuel 16:7, Proverbs 21:2, and Jeremiah 17:10. What do you observe about God's view of our hearts?

Image Management, New Testament Style

There's a group of people in the Bible who excelled at image management, believing it was their path to righteousness. The Pharisees were most concerned about how they looked to others. They were obvious when they fasted (Matthew 6:16). They prayed bold and loud prayers so everyone could hear them and be impressed. And they followed all the rules. They were quite proud of their ability to live clean and "holy" lives. They wanted everyone to believe they were flawless.

I've thought (too often) that if I could just get it all together, I wouldn't be braggy like those Pharisees. My goal wasn't to show off. I just wanted to stop stressing about my body. Life would be more comfortable and enjoyable if I could just rest in a place where I was happy with myself. *As soon as I love the way I look, I'll be free!*

What types of similar thoughts have you had?

This is why I struggle with seeing myself in pictures. It's an image issue. When I look at a photo that doesn't match the vision I have of my image, it unsettles me. *What if other people see the picture and have the same negative thoughts about me that I'm having? What if they think I look fat in this picture?*

What if they think that I look tired, unhealthy, out of shape, lazy, or unsuccessful? Fill in the word(s) you fear most here:

More Than an Image

Sure, we all get caught in less-than-flattering photos sometimes. But the reality is, my friends and family aren't shocked at how I look in pictures because they spend more time looking at me than I do! And let's be real, when we see ourselves in a group photo, most of us are more focused on how *we* look in that picture, not how others look.

Our struggle with photos encapsulates a larger issue. Too often, we dissect our image from the real us. The photo portrays my body, but I am not my image. Yes, the image looks like me. Others would say, "Oh, there's a picture of Heather. Let me tag her." *Oh, goodness. Does anyone like to be tagged?*

But that image is not *all* of me. It's only one aspect. **When I confuse who I am with my image, I objectify myself.** I see myself one-dimensionally, as a body only, and not as a whole person—with a mind, emotions, spirit, and soul. (We'll talk more about objectification soon.) At the heart of every struggle is the tension between who we are and who we want to be. It's the battle between an image we curate and our authentic self. Healing comes not through perfecting your image but through changing your perspective.

Work It Out

Why don't I like my image sometimes?

Are there images of me that I'm happy with?

Why do I feel happy with those images?

Am I more concerned about what I think of my image or what others think of my image?

What to Do if You Don't Like Yourself in Pictures

Here are a few quick tips if you find yourself spiraling after seeing yourself in a picture.

1. **Don't** overanalyze it. Don't stare. Nothing healthy comes from obsessing over it.
2. **Don't** compare your image with the image of others. Lighting, makeup, angles, and the photographer's expertise all play an important role in making models (and even "regular" women) look the way they do.
3. **Do** remember that the photo can't aptly capture your heart, your personality, or the fondness felt among you at that moment. It's just an image. It has no soul.
4. **Do** remember that God made you to be more than just an image. Even if you don't like what you reflect in pictures, when you reflect him in your life, his beauty will shine through you.

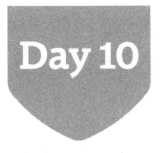

Ideal Image

What am I supposed to look like?

> I wish I didn't feel like there's a better version of me out there. I feel that way all the time.
>
> *Taylor Swift*

There's a chain of laser hair removal stores with the words "ideal" and "image" in their name. Their ads tout how their treatments can help me enjoy the summer because I'll look "hotter" in a swimsuit. *If I'd known that the secret to all my body problems was stubble-free armpits, I would have signed up decades ago!*

Now, there's nothing wrong with laser hair removal. It sounds delightful to never shave again! It's the constant stream of guarantees of what will make our life better that frustrates and demoralizes us. They're rampant on magazine covers; Instagram ads break into our feeds and commercials interrupt HGTV. They subtly convince us that if our lives looked more like these ideal images, then we'd be happier.

But the real promise marketers sell is bigger than shiny hair, smooth skin, and a whittled waist. They lure us with the promise of freedom, a story of rescue. **Ideal images offer us a path of deliverance from the pain of an imperfect life.**

Unlike Domino's pizza, the ideal image will never deliver. Intellectually, we get it. Deliverance from life struggles *is* a lot to expect from laser hair removal. Yet piece by piece, we still hold hope that someday our self-improvement projects will be complete and life will feel different. How could it not be "better" once we've become our "best" selves? (We'll explore where this psychology comes from in a few days.)

Promises, Promises

I've been fooled by the promise of my ideal image. It's like when a time-share company calls to say you've won an all-expenses-paid trip to a resort in Mexico. You want to believe it's true, but there's always a four-hour, high-pressure presentation that makes you regret leaving home.

And that's the most important thing to recognize about the "ideal me." This vision—this ideal of my imagination—offers false salvation. It tells me that much of the struggle, toil, and pain of this life could be avoided if I just changed my body. It's as if peace and prosperity are sitting in the rafters of heaven, ready to pour over me as soon as I shed the pounds, get the procedure, or peak my physique.

We believe these promises because we long to be rescued. God put that desire inside us. We crave a before-and-after, a life makeover story. But in pursuing this kind of temporary salvation, we miss a huge spiritual truth. Even after growing up in church and attending Christian schools, I didn't fully grasp this truth until my mid-thirties. Then it changed my life forever. Are you ready to hear it? **Our ideals always become our idols.**[1]

If It's on a Pedestal, It Could Be an Idol

Chasing the ideal body with the hope that it will save me from earthly struggle is idolatry. It's crazy to think about, but it's the same kind of bowing-down-to-a-golden-calf idol worship we see in Scripture.

Now, let me assure you, I had *no* idea I was an idolator. In fact, I was quite certain I'd never broken the first commandment. Who would be so foolish as to believe a fake god would help them? Burning sacrifices to a farm animal made of gold earrings? *Those people in the Old Testament must not have been very smart.*

And yet, I see it all differently now. My ideal image sits like a shiny specimen on a pedestal in my mind. Every day I assess my standing with her. She beckons me to be like her. If I fall short, I fail.

---

1. I originally used this line in my book *The Burden of Better.*

How does framing your ideals as idols change the way you think of them?

The Ideal Me

See if you can relate to my ideal idol. The ideal me is stylishly dressed in a much smaller size. She's so confident, she doesn't need to change clothes five times before leaving the house. She's a loving wife, a calm and patient parent—just the right mix of rules enforcement and fun mom. The ideal me doesn't read into the tone of benign statements from friends. Neither does she question it when they don't immediately reply to text messages. She's the picture of discipline, never missing a workout. Neither would she ever go back and eat three more cookies after vowing she'd only eat one. *She's a success story!*

But on bad hair days or when I feel extra bloated, each time my words come out wrong or I skip a workout or lose my temper with my kids—ideal me shows up to chastise. She pretends she's helping me stay on track. But like an evil stepmother, she keeps a running tally of all my mistakes and missteps.

Do you keep mental lists of ways you aren't measuring up? What's on these lists? What ideals for yourself have you clung to?

My Goals or His?

The ideal me is a blend of fiction, fantasy, and maybe a little delusion too. **I succumb to magical thinking and believe that I can find the right formula to let this "better me" come bubbling out.** This isn't biblical; it's mysticism. My ideal image is a creation—but not one of God's. She was formed in my imagination. Romans 1:25 explains this as a common challenge: "They exchanged the truth about God for a lie, and worshiped and served created things rather than the Creator—who is forever praised." The pursuit of the ideal me leads me to bow to golden calves.

Work It Out

Read 2 Corinthians 10:5–6 in the King James version first, then in two more modern translations. What does the Bible say about these versions of ourselves we imagine? How are our ideals imaginations?

Read Exodus 20. Why do you think idols are mentioned in the first commandment?

Act

What do I believe looking more like my ideal image would do for my life?

How does my ideal image match God's image for my life?

How does it distract from God's plan for me?

Who Told You That?

Identifying voices that influenced our struggle

> If only our eyes saw souls instead of bodies, how very different our ideals of beauty would be.
>
> *Anonymous*

I coach my clients in an exercise where they identify the specific images they idealize most. My client Kat was surprised by her results. Her ideal image was an obscure fitness influencer she followed on Instagram. *Where did this come from? Who told her she should look like this woman?*

Her parents weren't fitness fanatics. She couldn't even remember why she joined CrossFit. Of course, she secretly hoped the intense exercise would take the pressure off her dieting. With daily workouts, Kat reasoned, she'd be freer to eat what she wanted, when she wanted. But the further immersed she became in the gym culture, the more she began to obsess over clean eating.

Kat knew she wasn't in a good place. She would've never called it an eating disorder until the day her son ate her last protein bar. He didn't throw away the box, so she didn't know it was empty. Kat returned home from a workout, ravenous and ready to scarf down the chewy sustenance she'd dreamt about all afternoon. But it was gone! She was livid. Her response seemed grossly mismatched to her son's offense. Kat's overreaction opened her husband's eyes. While all outward signs signaled that his wife was thriving on the path to optimal health, there was something deeply wrong.

As Kat and I explored her ideal image, we talked about how she believed looking more like that fitness influencer would improve her life. Kat waffled between easy answers and bewilderment. Why did she feel so driven to improve her body? She fought embarrassment as she shared hidden beliefs and expectations. She had a loving husband and great children. She convinced herself she was pursuing health for them! But deep down, she knew that there was nothing healthy about this obsession. Why did she "need" her body to be more toned? Why did she chase that fitness ideal so hard? Who told her this was the body she needed?

Who Said You're Naked?

Way back in Genesis, after Adam and Eve ate from the one forbidden tree in the garden, they felt something they'd never felt before: shame. In Genesis 3:11, God asked the world's first couple how they knew they were naked. Then he asked them if they'd done that one thing he told them not to do. Instead of confessing, they blame-shifted and squirmed behind their fig leaves.

Our ideal images hold power over us through their ability to shame us. We believe their definitions of the truth—that life *would* be better if we just had a better body. We long for relief from the pressure, so we chase. The circular reasoning sounds something like this: *If I could just lose the weight, then at least I'd feel free from this constant nagging pressure to lose weight.*

Shame makes us desperate for an escape. But when the relief doesn't come as we hope, the shame multiplies. Can you relate?

A Truly Ideal Image

We'll explore shame more soon, but today let's talk about what our *true* ideal image is. We were made in God's image. So technically, he is our ideal. And yet, these other ideal images—the ones we've adopted from culture and made our very own—seem to have *more* power and influence in our lives. Of course, no one *actually* holds more power than the God of the universe! But like it did for Adam and Eve, sin separates us from God, and then shame makes us want to hide from him (and others).

Until this point, Adam and Eve had not felt the need to hide their bodies. But after eating the fruit, they had the ability to discern for themselves the difference between good and evil. In other words, they could make judgments about what they believed was good or bad, apart from what God had told them. These judgments extended to beliefs about their bodies.

Then Adam and Eve felt vulnerable. No longer covered by God's glory and protection, they became aware of their nakedness and decided it must be wrong. *Better cover these bodies up, fast!* Seems Eve is the first woman recorded in history with body image issues. Consider how strange that is, given that she was the only woman on the planet!

Through the days of Creation, earlier in the book of Genesis, we read that "God saw that it was good." *Good* here can be translated as *fitting* or even *beautiful*. God designed our images to be a lovely reflection of his glory. But when we pursue other images or fall prey to the temptation to decide *for ourselves* what is good and what is not good, we doubt God's sovereignty.

Read Genesis 3. What do you observe in this part of Adam and Eve's story?

Who Told You to Be Better?

Let's dig deeper into the question God asks Adam and Eve, and apply it to our struggle: Who told you that you're naked? Okay, I know you're likely wearing clothes right now. *Most of us with body image issues tend to prefer them.* But metaphorically, why do you feel so exposed?

Why do you believe that your body needs to be different?

Who told you that you should be ashamed of your body? Who insinuated or told you directly that your body should be "better"?

We didn't concoct our ideals in seclusion. We've each been influenced in more ways than we know by family members, friends, co-workers, media, and even music. Though we'd rather blame marketers, my clients are more likely to hear their mom's or dad's voice when they stare in the mirror and criticize their looks. Chances are there's someone—or a list of someones—whose words about your body have attached to your identity.

It could be that no words were ever said about your body, but you acutely observed words spoken over the bodies of others and determined to never be the target of that type of disapproval. Rejections of both kinds scar our body image and disrupt our relationship with food, exercise, and our emotions. **Everything we've been told about who we are connects to both the image we've created of ourselves and to our ideal image—who we believe we should be.**

This exercise is not to blame. Though it's tempting, faulting that cruel clique, the hurtful parent, or the guy who never asked you out (*he wasn't right for you anyway, trust me*) would miss the root of the problem.

The external bully morphs into an internal bully as we adopt the lies spoken over us and mesh them into our thoughts. Think of your lies list you started on Day 4 and where the lies originated. Who said them? Know it's okay to keep these discoveries to yourself as you work through them, especially if you're still in a relationship with them.

Determining where some of the thought patterns and beliefs about our bodies started helps us sort through the why behind our struggle. You didn't just decide to be unhappy with your body one day. But remember, just because someone influential sprinkled harmful seeds in your heart doesn't mean you have to continue to tend to the poisonous plants that have grown.

Work It Out

Write on this mirror below what's been said about your image and who said it. These words may be both positive and negative. Any words that come to mind that you believe describe your body image can be included.

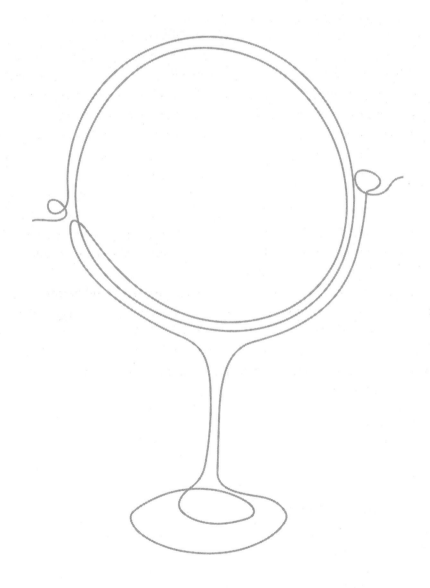

Act

Blot It Out

On a notecard, write a list of specific ways you were shamed, teased, or influenced into believing your body wasn't acceptable.

Daily pray over the list, asking God to help you forgive the person who shamed you, until you start to feel a release from the attachment of the memory. As you do, black out the memory on the notecard so it can no longer be read. **Keep praying daily until each item on your list is blotted out.**

Note: If the attachment is too strong or triggers traumatic memories, consider working with a Christian counselor for additional support.

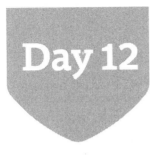

Image Wearers or Image Bearers

What does God expect of our image?

> Fashion fades, style is eternal.
>
> *Yves Saint Laurent*

I have video of my youngest son, Drew, as a four-year-old, running in and out of the room, changing identities. "I Cap'in 'Merica!" he proclaimed, wearing a suit with Poly-fil muscles and carrying a shield. Then he raced away to grab another superhero tool and mask. Within minutes, that boy cycled through a collection of costumes, changing identities as quickly as he could get them on and off.

Of course, the costumes didn't really make him an Avenger. No matter how many times he called himself Spiderman, I knew he wasn't equipped to scale walls or shoot webs. He *wore* the superhero image, but he didn't *bear* the image.

Similarly, culture confuses our image-wearing and our image-bearing. There are many images out there luring us to wear them. *Follow my plan to get a body like mine!* Yet transforming our bodies and changing them to keep up with the Kardashians or whoever is hottest on TikTok are ways we put on the images of others. Even if I plump my lips, add hair extensions, and get a few strategic augmentation surgeries in an attempt to look like the "ideal body" of the season, chances are I'll only look like an overly operated-on version of me.

Bearing God's Image

Though I feel the pressure to wear all sorts of images, God's expectations of my image seem significantly more reasonable than mine. Let's revisit Genesis 1:27, where we read how God made humankind in his own image. In the previous verses, the Bible says God made animals and sea creatures like "their kind." But when God creates people, the language changes to say we're made in God's image. We are not the same kind as Dachshunds or dolphins. We are the same kind as God.

We bear God's image. It's not something we have to put on each day or get surgery to replicate. Instead, we have aspects of him beaming from our insides out. Bearing his image means we show all of creation who God is through our existence.

In His Image

The further I try to separate myself from the original (God) or satisfy myself in my image apart from him, the more frustrated I feel. This pull to be an image *apart* from God—to reflect my own wants and desires instead of his—is how our original image became fractured. Adam and Eve's sin marred our perfect image. Jesus came and lived the perfect life in the image of God. Through his death and resurrection, we can be reconnected with the one whose image we bear.

Idols blur the lines, confusing us into believing they offer what we need to restore our image. They claim to help us "fix" all that we feel is broken about us. **They convince us that we can re-create our bodies into our own masterpieces and that we'll be happy with how they turn out.** But idols aren't originals. They don't have that kind of power. They're just God copycats, and that's where the trouble begins. Idols can't create.

Idols of Image

Idols convince us to become image wearers instead of image bearers. Though we may claim to be glad we're made in God's image, secretly, I know I've been prouder of ways I resembled my favorite celebrity. *Yikes!*

Truth is, even if we each woke up tomorrow morning looking just like that woman we idolize—we wouldn't be satisfied. We'd feel like a fake or a replica. Others may affirm this lack of originality. *You're so pretty. You look just like . . .*

Image-wearing confuses our value, identity, and worth as we layer on aspects of images we admire. We were created to bear God's image. It's a perfect fit. Wearing others' images will always feel as awkward as trying on last year's shorts in the middle of winter.

Thriving in God's assignment to bear his image makes me feel genuine and alive. Without changing my body, I can show others his love, mercy, goodness, and compassion. Are you trying to awkwardly wear someone else's image when all God asks is that you bear his?

Work It Out

In what ways have you tried to "wear" the images of others?

What aspects of your ideal image have you tried to force your own body to match?

How does the illustration of a young child putting on a costume affect the way you see yourself trying to match an ideal image?

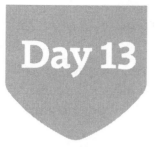

The Image Idol

A history

> They abandoned the LORD to serve Baal and the images of Ashtoreth.
>
> *Judges 2:13 NLT*

The Old Testament's most famous sister wives—Rachel and Leah—certainly had some image issues to work through. As you may remember, Rachel was beautiful but struggled to have babies. Meanwhile, Leah desperately hoped motherhood would earn her the love of her husband and help her feel secure. Let's look closer at a quirky detail toward the end of their story.

Jacob decides it's time to flee from his boss-turned-father-in-law. He secretly packs up the wives and kids and departs. Grandpa Laban isn't happy about not kissing his daughters and grandkids good-bye (or so he says), so he chases after them. When he finds them, he makes an interesting accusation. He claims they stole the household idols (Genesis 31).

Jacob thought this was absurd. By this time, he and God had already had their wrestling match. Certain that no one from his household had stolen the idols, he told Laban to check everyone's possessions. Anyone caught carrying them should be killed.

Laban never found those idols. But that doesn't mean they weren't stolen. Scripture tells us that Rachel, Jacob's favorite wife, sat on them. She told Dad she had her period so she wouldn't have to get up.

Why did Rachel want these idols, anyway? I picture them as little statues—knickknacks. *Why bother?* It's easier to understand once you dig into the history.

In that era, household gods were often idols of fertility. Ancient people believed that they needed these idols to have babies—the ultimate status symbol of the age. And what did dear Rachel want more than anything? Babies! *Fertile* was their version of *hot*.

You see, image idols are nothing new. In Ancient Greece, she was called Aphrodite; in Ancient Rome, they called her Venus. The goddess of love, sex, fertility, and beauty had long hair and curves everywhere. Mythology holds that men couldn't help but fall in love with her. Aphrodite was the ultimate symbol of sexual prowess.

The city of Corinth—which you may recognize from the New Testament—was a well-known center for the worship of Aphrodite. In Paul's letters to the Corinthians, he mentions their sexual perversion. Paul also spells out what real love looks like in 1 Corinthians 13. Thinking about this famous passage in the context of a culture where love was defined in sexual terms gives it even more meaning. **Defining love sexually isn't foreign to the modern world, is it?**

But let's go back even further. Rachel and Leah lived in Ancient Mesopotamia before Greece and Rome were even founded. The ancient world had a precursor to these idols named Ishtar. She was the goddess of war and sexual love—characterized as young, beautiful, and impulsive. Even though fertility was a status symbol, Ishtar was never portrayed as a helpmate or mother.[1] Instead, even four millennia ago, a hypersexualized, superhero type of beauty beckoned women to be like her.

In Canaanite culture, they called the goddess *Ashtoreth*. Hebrew scholars believe this is a blending of the Greek name *Astarte* and the Hebrew word for shame, *boshet*. The Israelites (Jacob's family and ancestors) had great disdain for her, so *Ashtoreth* became a general term the Hebrews used when referencing goddesses and paganism.[2]

Throughout the Old Testament we can spot references to this idol. In 2 Kings 23, Josiah destroyed the cult places of Ashtoreth. In Jeremiah 44, the people burned offerings and poured libations to the "Queen of Heaven"—Ashtoreth.

1. Encyclopedia Britannica, "Ishtar," accessed May 2023, https://www.britannica.com/topic/Ishtar-Mesopotamian-goddess.
2. Encyclopedia Britannica, "Astarte," accessed May 2023, https://www.britannica.com/topic/Astarte-ancient-deity.

In Ezekiel 8:5, God shows the prophet a vision of this goddess who invokes the people's jealousy. The idol of this shapely vixen sits at the entrance to the temple, captivating worship to her image and away from God.

In Judges 2:13 and 10:6–7, we read more about Israel's struggle with idol worship. Judges 2:13 (NLT) reads, "They abandoned the LORD to serve Baal and the images of Ashtoreth." Serving Baal would be the ancient equivalent of one serving money. But to worship the images of Ashtoreth was to worship beauty, sensuality, fertility, and sex.

How do you see beauty, sensuality, fertility, and sex worshiped in our culture?

Have you ever connected idol worship with body image issues? How do you think they may connect?

Jesus Plus

I don't know where Rachel's heart was in her relationship with God, but I have empathy for her struggle. I've operated, too often, as if I needed Jesus to get me into heaven and other things to rescue me on earth. Jesus *plus* weight loss. Jesus *plus* clearer skin. Jesus *plus* flatter abs. I subtly bowed to our culture's worship of the ideal body as a path to peace and rest from the chaos of life. *If I could just look like her, then I would be free, filled with joy.* But idols never keep their promises. Only God can be trusted to do that.

This beckoning to beautify what we deem beastly about our bodies is truly a tale as old as time. The beauty goddess has tempted women to follow her since the fall of man. She promises love, approval, and affection—but she can only define these terms within the limits of her powers.

Just like real beauty doesn't look like an ancient goddess, real love doesn't look like admiration for your curves or facial symmetry. Instead, it looks like patience, kindness, and long-suffering commitment. Real love is what Jesus displayed for us on the cross. God wants us to be imitators of Jesus with beautiful hearts.

Work It Out

Read the verses referenced today about the worship of these goddesses. In what ways do you observe our culture worshiping image?

How was it helpful to understand the history of this idol worship?

Read Galatians 4:8–9. What do false gods/idols do to us?

Read 1 Samuel 7:3–4 and 1 John 5:21. What does the Bible tell us to do when it comes to idols in both the Old Testament and the New Testament?

Act

Pause and read 1 Corinthians 13:4–8.

Why do you think Paul spells out the characteristics of real love to the people of Corinth?

How does culture's definition of these words contrast with Scripture?

How does the context of their worship of Aphrodite—the goddess of sex and beauty—change the way you read this passage?

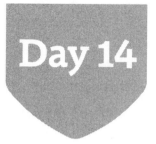

Day 14

Lessons from the Sneetches

Identifying your image idols

> Now, the Star-Belly Sneetches had bellies with stars. The Plain-Belly Sneetches had none upon thars....
>
> *Dr. Seuss*

The 1961 Dr. Seuss classic *The Sneetches* was written to teach children a lesson about discrimination. But it also teaches a relevant lesson on body image. There were two different Sneetch body types. When those Sneetches started comparing themselves to each other on the beaches (*Who would ever do that?*), the plain-bellies felt unhappy with their starless bodies.

Those Sneetches were in a real bind until an enterprising huckster named Sylvester McMonkey McBean invented a way for them to "fix" their bodies. *Star implants, anyone?*

But the star-bellied Sneetches no longer felt special. Everyone had stars now. Never fear. Sylvester offered a new "beach body" plan to shed those stars. Star-bellied Sneetches lined up for laser star removal.

The cycle continued. The Sneetches keep gaining and losing their stars, and there's only one person who benefitted through the whole process: Sylvester McMonkey McBean. He drives off with a truckload of cash. Here's how their story concludes: "I'm quite happy to say that the Sneetches got really quite smart on that day, the day they decided that Sneetches are Sneetches and no kind of Sneetch is the best on the beaches."[1]

---

1. Dr. Seuss, *The Sneetches and Other Stories* (New York: Random House, 1961), 24.

Objectification

There's a sneaky distinction between our true selves and our ideal selves, and that is *objectification*.

When we see the body as malleable, measurable, and controllable, we're more likely to view our bodies as objects.[2] **By becoming observers of our bodies instead of inhabitants of them, we see our value through our usefulness to others—including sexual desirability.** From shame to anxiety, depression to eating disorders, the consequences of seeing our body as a commodity are severe.[3]

Write your own definition of objectification. Who do you tend to objectify? What kinds of messages do you observe in our culture about objectification? Is it acceptable, desirable, disgusting, or a little of everything?

Who Loves Worship?

Our culture loves the "perfect" body, yet that standard of "excellence" keeps changing. In the late 1960s, a model named Twiggy made girls long for skinnier figures. Similarly, when I was a fitness instructor in the early 2000s, everyone longed to work the roundness of their butts "off." Then Meghan Trainor taught us to be "all about that bass." Now you can pay for butt implants or wear shapewear that gives you a fuller bottom. "Perfect" can only be defined inside a precise place and time, making it completely amorphous.

Some seek sexualized images of the "perfect" woman that requires nothing from them. They can take from her in their imaginations and not give anything in return. When they lust, they worship.

Others worship the "perfect" image in different ways. We covet her abs, butt, or arms. We long to have her perfect hair, her perfect smile, or her perky breasts. **Culture teaches that anyone who meets its standard of beauty truly deserves our worship.** Think about how we treat celebrities. We stalk them on socials.

---

2. R. M. Calogero, "Objectification Theory, Self-Objectification, and Body Image," *Encyclopedia of Body Image and Human Appearance* vol. 2 (Academic Press, 2012), 574–80, https://doi.org/10.1016/b978-0-12-384925-0.00091-2.

3. Melissa Grey, "The Influences of Identities and Social Connectedness on Self-Objectification," (master's thesis, Eastern Michigan University, 2007), https://commons.emich.edu/cgi/viewcontent.cgi?article=1140&context=theses.

We buy the magazine because their photo is on it. We go to the movies to see more. We follow out of a desire to learn from their greatness or because we're just curious about how people "like that" live. And if we're honest, we may spend more time worshiping our celeb idols than we do Jesus. *Lord, help us!*

God did create beauty. He designed our human eyes to appreciate it and our human hearts to desire it. But he never intended for us to worship beauty—at least not the earthly kind.

What does the word worship *mean to you?*

Isaiah 42:8 reminds us that God won't share his glory with idols. Why is this important to remember?

The Best on the Beaches

In addition to misplacing our worship, objectification opens the door for both envy and discrimination. When we, like the Sneetches, decide who looks best on the beaches, are we not claiming one body size or shape as superior to the others? How is this different from asserting a superior hair color, eye color, or race?

We're called to love everyone. Whether they sparkle with that "star quality" or they look like they're suffering to make it through their day, Jesus says to love them. Show kindness. Act justly. Be merciful. Give them grace. Don't cast judgments on their appearance (see John 7:24).

By observing the body types I'm most tempted to worship, I learn where I'm still stuck in my own wrong thinking. When I objectify others, I fail to love well. When I compare myself to others, I have only two options—pride that comes with feeling like I'm doing "better" than they are, or shame that follows the feeling that I'm not keeping up. The image idol blinds me into believing that because someone else has the body I long for, they also have the freedom and rest I desire. But idols always lie. And worshiping an idol will never deliver the body image freedom I long for.

Work It Out

Identifying Your Idols Exercise

What are some things you've worshiped in your life?

Idols can be good things like family, children, career, health, or even success. There's nothing wrong with these things. But when one demands and dominates your thoughts, time, finances, fantasies, emotions, or fears, your relationship may have turned to worship.

In today's exercise, you'll consider a list of various idols that tempt us. You'll have an opportunity to circle the idols that may be a challenge for you. As you consider the idol options in the list, think about these questions:

What do you spend the most time thinking about?

What do you freely spend money on?

What do you fear losing the most?

What do you believe will bring the most satisfaction?

What do you notice and admire most about others (e.g., their bodies, their wealth, their success, their discipline, their food choices, their marital status . . .)?

What types of mistakes frustrate you the most (e.g., missing a workout, being late for work, missing a friend's birthday, feeling like you're a "bad" spouse, etc.)?

Note: Food can also be an idol, but our physical need for food, along with a physiologically driven hyper-focus on food that can be present for those with a history of disordered eating, makes it confusing to identify. For women with body image issues, food is not often a primary idol. Rather, a strong desire to recognize food as an idol could indicate eating disorder/disordered eating thought patterns.

Some Idol Options

Idols can take various forms and names. Even the body image idol can be very different from person to person. But here are some idols to consider based on your answers above. Circle the ones that apply to you:

Body image idol	Beauty idol	Productivity idol
Marriage idol	Thinness idol	Health idol
Money idol	Family idol	Exercise idol
Success idol	Perfection idol	Friendship idol
Personality idol	Love/Approval idol	Sex idol
Romance idol	Moral virtue idol	Intelligence idol
Political cause idol	Power idol	Fame idol
Control idol	Comfort idol	

Act

Read Daniel 3. It's the story of three brave men—Shadrach, Meshach, and Abednego—who refused to bow down to a ninety-foot-tall idol. God rewarded their faithfulness, and everyone witnessed God's power as he spared them from even the slightest singe in the fiery furnace.

Because culturally we aren't asked to physically bow to gold images, it's sometimes hard to visualize how our modern-day idols beckon our worship. **Take a few minutes and draw on a separate sheet of paper what a few of your idols circled above would look like as statues.** Even if you're not an artist, you can still put symbols or words on a pedestal to help visualize it.

Consider the following as you draw: What would your idol be shaped like? What would your idol hold to symbolize its promises or virtue? Would there be words or an inscription on the idol that it uses to "inspire" you?

Place these images on your mirror or somewhere you can see them daily. Spend a few seconds each day staring at the images you've created and saying out loud that you will not bow. Pray daily that God will help you see when you're tempted to bow and help *you* escape the fire of not conforming to the idols of this world.

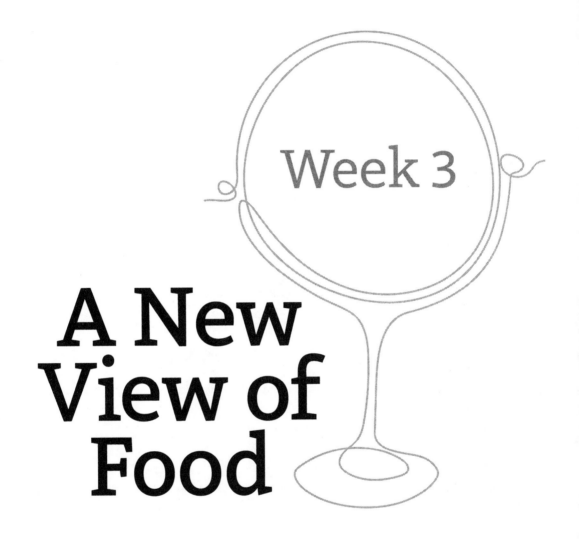

Week 3

A New View of Food

Day 15

The Con of Diet Culture

What have you believed?

> The true con artist doesn't force us to do anything; he makes us complicit in our own undoing. He doesn't steal. We give. He doesn't have to threaten us. We supply the story ourselves. We believe because we want to, not because anyone made us.
>
> *Maria Konnikova*

The bad guy was always easy to spot on shows like *Dateline*. He said the right things. He did the right things. But it was clear to everyone watching that he was a con artist. *I'd never fall for anything like that.* Or so I believed. . . .

But there's an effort to swindle men and women that I was subject to for decades. It stole copious amounts of my money and time, and it eventually caused me health issues. What was this fraudulent creep? It's called diet culture, and it has overcomplicated our relationship with food.

Relationship with food? Have we ever even paused to think about how bizarre it is to characterize food in this way? But diet culture has taught us many strange customs as a part of its con.

Diet culture is an umbrella term that author Christy Harrison defines as "a system of beliefs that worships thinness and equates it to health and moral virtue . . . promotes weight loss as a means of attaining higher status . . . demonizes certain ways of eating while elevating others . . . [and] oppresses people who don't match up with its supposed picture of 'health'..."[1] Understand, diet culture isn't just about weight loss. Many companies selling clearer skin, age-less beauty, toning tools, and even better health have benefited from the pronounced teaching and broad acceptance of this scam.

We've worked through the spiritual dimensions of body image issues. Now we'll take a practical look at how idolatry, worship, objectification, and related concepts are taught, promoted, and endorsed everywhere we look. Let's examine how these messages impact how we view food and our bodies.

Diet culture is so widely accepted it's almost sacrilegious not to believe that its claims are true. Diet culture teaches us what foods to eat and which to avoid, it dictates what body parts we should be slimming and which are "sexier" when left full, and it decides for us what's "healthy." Even your doctor may subscribe to its newsletters.

Maybe instead of trying to lose weight, you've tried to gain weight. Or perhaps you've struggled with your height or the appearance of your skin. **After years of coaching, I've recognized that most who struggle with body image issues also, at some level, struggle with food.** One study of American women showed 74.5 percent of women had concerns about their shape that affected their happiness. Of this group, 10 percent met the criteria for an identifiable eating disorder, while an additional 31 percent fit the criteria for an unspecified eating disorder. Two-thirds of the entire sample reported they were currently trying to lose weight and that weight-loss-related behaviors consumed their time and energy.[2]

I Know Victoria's Secret

There's a song on pop radio that unveils how a certain lingerie store may promulgate body issues. The witty punchline in the chorus points to a man in Ohio being behind it all. Hopefully the revelation helps women understand the contrived nature of the beauty standards set before us. But I don't think he should

---

1. Christy Harrison, "What Is Diet Culture?" August 10, 2018, https://christyharrison.com/blog/what-is-diet-culture.
2. L. Reba-Harrelson, A. Von Holle, R. M. Hamer, R. Swann, M. L. Reyes, C. M. Bulik, "Patterns and Prevalence of Disordered Eating and Weight Control Behaviors in Women Ages 25–45," *Eating and Weight Disorders* 14, no. 4, July 27, 2013, https://link.springer.com/article/10.1007/BF03325116#citeas.

shoulder the blame alone. More broadly, diet culture exploits us. **It leads us to believe that we're "irreparably broken" if we don't match the ideal.**[3] Then it capitalizes on our desire to be rescued from the pain of our perceived flaws, selling us the chance to be healed, fixed, whole, and beautiful.

Of course, anyone in a "better" body can tell you that she still struggles. Models (even "Angels") wrestle body image issues.[4] But we compartmentalize those truths in our quest for relief. If there's even the slightest chance the next plan could lead me out of body image woe, I can't afford to miss it.

Afford may be the wrong word. Consumers spend about seventy billion dollars annually on diets, exercise programs, and the peddled goods of diet culture.[5] The industry has mushroomed in the past few decades. Some estimate the average person will spend more than $112,000 dollars in a lifetime on diet and fitness programs.[6] *No judgment here.* I've happily handed over my credit card to "invest" in body improvement.

Body Change Can't Rescue Us

You're not bad if you desire the diet that will "fix it all"! Neither is there any reason to feel shame if you've tried all the plans and have a cabinet full of supplements and exercise gear that never worked for you. *I'm right there with you, my friend.*

Diet culture's lies seemed credible. Who doesn't want to transform from a "before" to an "after"? Who doesn't want a guarantee of better health? But no one running after diet culture's con finds the peace it promises. Even if the plan offers success, you must keep striving to maintain that size and shape, pressured by the fear of losing it. If you meet your goal, you don't win everlasting freedom. Instead, you go on their "maintenance" plan. Hard-earned results disappear if you "let your guard down." **There's no rest in an "after" picture. Often, the pressure to maintain becomes greater than the original pressure to lose.**

3. Christy Harrison, *Anti-Diet* (New York: Little, Brown and Company, 2019), 95.

4. Jo Abi, "Australian Victoria's Secret Model No Longer Fits into Runway Bra," Honey, https://honey.nine.com.au/latest/victorias-secret-model-talks-about-body-image-issues/81987ba5-4783-4cc9-8fdc-93ff9db0244b.

5. Allison Lau, "The Rise of Fad Diets," CNBC, January 11, 2021, https://www.cnbc.com/video/2021/01/11/how-dieting-became-a-71-billion-industry-from-atkins-and-paleo-to-noom.html.

6. Arabella Ogilvie, "How Much Do Americans Spend on Health and Fitness? Survey Results Revealed," MYPROTEIN, January 3, 2020, https://us.myprotein.com/thezone/training/much-americans-spend-health-fitness-survey-results-revealed.

I'm also pretty sure there are no crowns in heaven for reaching your goal weight. But it's hard to live like this is true. For me, pursuing a better body felt like a more natural and comfortable quest than pursuing Christlikeness. Plus, it came with instant recognition and rewards. "Oh, Heather! Have you lost weight? You look great!" No one's ever stopped me in Target to tell me they see the fruit of the Spirit blooming in my life.

Similarly, diet culture's pervasiveness gaslights us. To question its claims is akin to questioning gravity or the roundness of the earth. It's so ingrained that as you read the following chapters, you may even feel a certain zeal for its principles rise up within you. I only ask that you approach this topic with curiosity. Could it be that not all is as it seems when it comes to how we've been taught to think about food? When we uncover diet culture's con, it becomes even easier to see our body image struggles as matters of the heart, not the body.

Work It Out

What are your main takeaways from today?

How does the language about diet culture "saving us" strike you?

In what ways have you accepted diet culture's message that you are "irreparably broken" if you don't match culture's ideal?

Act

I spent most of my life trying to hide my own brokenness, believing that if others saw me as broken, they would see me as weak or undesirable. But as Christians, we can embrace both our brokenness and a cure for that brokenness in Jesus. Diet culture can't heal brokenness, but God can. **Fill in the blanks to this prayer today.**

Prayer to Embrace the Cure for Our Brokenness

Dear Heavenly Father,
    You know the ways I feel broken. You know how I stress over _____

and worry over _____

and feel shame over _____

_____ .

Today, help me to remember that my brokenness is part of my humanness, not something I must be ashamed or afraid of. Give me grace to look to you to heal my brokenness. I confess I've tried to cover my brokenness through _____

_____ .

But today I boldly proclaim that Jesus is the only cure to what ails me.
In Jesus's name, Amen.

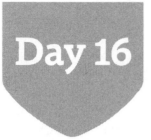

Day 16

The Religion of Diet Culture

What do we worship?

> If we are not deliberately thinking about our culture and our context, we will be conformed to it without ever knowing.
>
> *Tim Keller*

Yesterday we talked about how diet culture schemes ways to steal our money and our time. Today let's look at the ways diet culture diverts our worship. Examining the impact of popular culture on our lives demonstrates how powerful its influence can be.

At age nine, my daughter Katie—homeschooled with no access to the internet at the time—determined her favorite color was teal. Weeks later, I noticed teal was *the* color of the season. Somehow, she'd absorbed the subtle messages of pop culture. I still don't know how she learned teal was cool.

Diet culture possesses this same saturation power. Whatever the enemy foods are, most know them. Every influencer seems to read the same script, so we assume there's magic in this new way of eating. Even our pastors make quips about cutting carbs or following diet culture rules. Food labels follow trends to remind you that eggs are "gluten-free" and bread is "plant-based." Grocery stores arrange prominent displays with the items most likely to be on your new plan. It's not conspiracy theory—diet culture markets to us from every angle.

The word *culture* comes from the Latin root *cult*, meaning cultivated or worshiped. Cults are groups of people who may do strange things out of devotion to a person or a cause. Like-minded worship brings cult members together. Likewise, unified worship keeps diet culture thriving. You're likely not joining a cult when you sign up for a weight loss plan, of course. But if we're not careful, our hearts *can* be led astray to worship body transformation.

Pause and consider this question: How have you been influenced by diet culture's messages about food and your body?

An Alternative Religion

Years ago, God graciously showed me how I'd bought into the "cult" of diet culture. My language, habits, doctrine, beliefs, and values were influenced more heavily by its teaching than by the Bible. I confessed to being a Christian first, but in practice, I was more interested in following food and exercise rules as my real path to lasting freedom. **I tried to live straddling the fence—I believed God had saved me for eternity, but "bettering" myself was the rescue I needed for now.**

Though there are no food rules in the New Testament, I lived by the lie that eating clean, unprocessed foods was a more righteous way to live. Avoiding the "bad food" equaled holiness, and spiritual discipline felt connected to starving your body to look thinner. Defeating the flesh meant not giving in to food cravings, and spiritual warfare happened when I stared at the ice cream in the freezer.

My faith came by believing that results I could not see would someday come. My works? Those were tracked by MyFitnessPal and closing rings on my Apple Watch. **Freedom and peace would arrive when I reached my body goals.** And my sanctification process encompassed carefully following the plan. At night, I felt more condemnation and shame around breaking food rules than I felt conviction over my envy, pride, or idolatry. I confessed the off-plan foods I ate or workouts I skipped to friends more than I confessed my real sins to Jesus.

The Weigh Down

Sadly, there were times when even the church seemed to endorse my twisted faith. Though I never dabbled specifically in Christian weight loss plans, I remember hearing the story of David and Goliath taught as a battle between me and my weight loss goals. At the intersection of the church and diet culture sat a woman named Gwen Shamblin. She founded the Weigh Down Workshop in the mid-1980s.[7] By all accounts, she started in a healthy place. As a dietitian, Gwen saw how diets failed people and instead encouraged women to listen to their bodies to eat more intuitively. But somewhere along the path, Gwen shifted from the worship of Jesus to the worship of food rules and thinness. In *The Way Down*, a documentary that chronicles strange and cult-like behaviors at her "church," you overhear Shamblin finishing a demonstration to a crowd by saying something like, "This is how to avoid eating at Thanksgiving dinner." Witnesses claim they were only allowed a certain number of bites of food each day in the high-control atmosphere.[8] The god of their "church" was not the God of the Bible but the god of diet culture.

Romans 14:17 tells us that the kingdom of heaven isn't about eating and drinking. Look up this verse and write your thoughts here:

A System of Beliefs That Worships

Look at Christy Harrison's definition again. She's not making a case for diets as a false alternative to Jesus. Yet pay attention to the specific words she chose: "Diet culture is a *system of beliefs* that *worships* thinness and equates it to health and moral virtue . . ."[9] (emphasis added).

With language and promises similar to what we believe as Christians, there's only one way to distinguish the real from the fake—the cult from the Christian church. The practices, people, and procedures may look the same, but look at the object of their worship. **Diet culture worships beautiful bodies. Christians worship Jesus.**

7. Adrian Horton, "'This Is a Cult': Inside the Shocking Story of a Religious Weight-Loss Group," *The Guardian*, September 29, 2021, https://www.theguardian.com/tv-and-radio/2021/sep/29/gwen-shamblin-docuseries-the-way-down-remnant-fellowship.

8. *The Way Down: God, Greed, and the Cult of Gwen Shamblin*, directed by Marina Zenovich, 2021–2022, HBO Max.

9. Harrison, "What Is Diet Culture?"

Work It Out

Look at this chart and read the verses listed. In what ways have you believed or followed diets, fitness, or wellness plans with religious-like gusto? This doesn't mean it's bad to follow a plan or have someone lead you along a path to meet physical health goals. But if we let our plans rule our lives, look to them for rescue from our shame, or allow them to take a place of authority and worship only God should hold, we've ascribed to the religion of diet culture.

Religion of Diet Culture

Principle	Diet Culture's Definition	Bible's Definition
Faith	My faith is in this plan's ability to get me the body I want.	Romans 10:17 Ephesians 2:8 Hebrews 11
Righteousness	Righteousness is being "good" this week with eating and my exercise.	Romans 6:18 2 Timothy 2:22 2 Timothy 3:16 Proverbs 28:5
Hope	Hope is placed in someday getting the body I want, an "after" picture—then I'll find joy, peace, and rest.	1 Peter 1:13 Ephesians 1:18 Hebrews 10:23
Justice	If I eat "bad" things, then the scale or mirror will punish me. If I eat well, I'll get the results I deserve. I can be "just" if I try hard enough.	Psalm 37:28 Isaiah 30:18 Micah 6:8 Isaiah 61:8
Self-Control/ Defeating the Flesh	Temptation is about food not sin. Denying the flesh is about the ability to say no to certain foods.	Galatians 5:16–21 Romans 13:14 Ephesians 2:1–3
Holiness	Purity and holiness come from carefully monitoring what food and drink you put in your body. The standard of holiness is set by diet culture.	Psalm 96:9 Romans 6:19 Ephesians 4:23–24

How do you feel as you read this chart? Which of the nuanced religious promises of diet culture stand out to you most?

How have you felt the draw to worship ideas of culture or diet culture?

Act

If the concept of worship resonates with you, take a minute today to pause and confess to Jesus the ways you've misplaced worship. Like a loving father, he's ready to hear your repentance and forgive.

Watch this video for more information on the role of confession:
improvebodyimage.com/confession

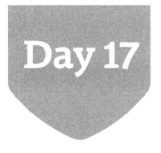

Day 17

Hunger Games

What happens when we're desperate?

In the Middle Ages, they had guillotines, stretch racks, whips and chains. Nowadays, we have a much more effective torture device called the bathroom scale.

Stephen Phillips

In 1728, writer Thomas Short observed in "A discourse concerning the causes and effects of corpulency" that "corpulent" people seemed to live near swamps. Thus, he brilliantly created a magnificent plan for staying slim. His first recommendation involved . . . you guessed it: moving away from swamps![1] *Silly, right?*

But what about eating half a grapefruit before every meal? Cabbage soup? Cotton balls? Yes, the last one was a real trend. In 2013, dieters ate cotton balls to help them feel full and lose weight. Because this leads to intestinal obstruction, the trend dissipated quickly (unlike the cotton balls!).[2]

Christy Harrison traces the history of diet culture back to a weight loss guru in Great Britain named William Banting. The year was 1862, and Banting wanted to drop some pounds. He found a doctor to help him and published a mini booklet on his success. The book skyrocketed to popularity, as did

1. Thomas Short, "A Discourse Concerning the Causes and Effects of Corpulency," Welcome Collection, https://wellcomecollection.org/works/ecvwka7u.
2. Melissa Wdowik, "The Long, Strange History of Dieting Fads," The Conversation, November 6, 2017, https://theconversation.com/the-long-strange-history-of-dieting-fads-82294.

scales for people to weigh themselves regularly. Previously, scales weren't a household item.

In the mid-1800s, weight gain was considered a normal part of aging, but by the early 1900s, physicians were on board with the idea that intentional weight loss was good. Bariatric surgeries came in the 1950s by a man named Howard Payne, who actually coined the term "morbid obesity" to make it look like unless people got his surgery, they would surely die.[3]

Weight Watchers, incorporated in 1963, enrolled five million people within the first five years. A decade later, Dr. Atkins taught us how to eat like they do in South Beach. Ten years after that, Jenny Craig threw her food rules in the ring and set up centers to help women across the country achieve their weight loss goals. I could spend the rest of this book listing for you the thousands of weight loss, fitness, and diet plans that have come and gone since the 1970s.

Diets Don't Work?

But here's data I've never heard in a weight loss commercial. In 1992, the National Institute of Health did research that concluded that diets don't work, and the majority of people who intentionally lost weight had regained most or all of it back within five years.[4] According to the *Washington Post*, by 1995, Americans were fatter than ever before. John P. Foreyt, a doctor from Baylor College of Medicine, contributed this sentiment to the article: "The more you diet, the worse it gets."[5]

Yet these headlines didn't stop anyone. A recent study shows we're still hoping to beat the odds. Forty-five million people in the United States alone try a new plan each year.[6] Another study showed that 45 percent of people globally are trying to lose weight.[7]

3. Harrison, *Anti-Diet*, 38.

4. NIH Technology Assessment Conference Panel, "Methods for Voluntary Weight Loss and Control," *Annals of Internal Medicine* 116, no. 11 (1992): 942, https://doi.org/10.7326/0003-4819-116-11-942.

5. Abigail Trafford, "Losing the Weight Battle," *The Washington Post*, February 7, 1995, https://www.washingtonpost.com/archive/lifestyle/wellness/1995/02/07/losing-the-weight-battle/da649449-bf3f-4bf1-a08f-f0999b0c9d31/.

6. Linda Searing, "The Big Number: 45 million Americans Go on a Diet Each Year," *The Washington Post*, January 1, 2018, https://www.washingtonpost.com/national/health-science/the-big-number-45-million-americans-go-on-a-diet-each-year/2017/12/29/04089aec-ebdd-11e7-b698-91d4e35920a3_story.html.

7. Pippa Bailey, Susan Purcell, Javier Calvar, and Alex Baverstock, "45% of People Globally are Trying to Lose Weight," IPSOS.com, January 18, 2021, https://www.ipsos.com/en/global-weight-and-actions.

Losing weight is hard. Keeping it off is close to impossible, even if you have expert help. A study that tracked contestants from *The Biggest Loser*, who learned eating and exercise strategies from the best, showed that contestants regained two-thirds of what they'd lost, on average, and a few became heavier than when they first appeared on the show.[8]

If you're dieting, trying to diet, or thinking about dieting—know you're not alone. I understand your desire to lose weight. But all this data begs the question: Why do we keep dieting if it doesn't work?

Pause and think about how many different plans you've tried to follow to change your body. Why would or wouldn't you consider another?

Worship of the body and appearance has existed since ancient times. But restricting food or food groups and measuring health by the number on the scale are more recent phenomena. More so, someone is benefiting from these ever-changing diet plans, and it's *not* the woman who struggles with body image issues. Sylvester McMonkey McBean from *The Sneetches* has many apprentices. Inventive "health" enthusiasts profit greatly by scaring society into believing that having the "wrong" body size is akin to being an outcast. Not following the popular food rules of the day puts you at risk of rejection, disapproval, and abandonment. **The pervasive message is that if you ever want to feel loved, you'd better work on your body. Fear is a powerful motivator for the diet industry.**

Yet a body that looks more runway ready can't promise you love, approval, or peace. All diets can offer is some sort of physical change. It may be weight loss, but it could be emotional or physical side effects that come with food restriction—like anxiety, hair loss, long-term digestive issues, or just a perpetually grumpy mood. Even if you diet to seek better health, weight loss alone can't promise you immunity from disease or suffering. Instead, diets offer a false sense of control. They convince us that following the plan will free us from body frustration. But no plan can keep that promise.

8. Erin Fothergill, et al., "Persistent Metabolic Adaptation 6 Years After 'The Biggest Loser' Competition," *Obesity* 24, no. 8 (August 2016): 1612–19, https://pubmed.ncbi.nlm.nih.gov/27136388/.

On a scale of 1–10, how desperate have you felt for the change a new plan promises?

1 · · · · · · · · 2 · · · · · · · · 3 · · · · · · · · 4 · · · · · · · · 5 · · · · · · · · 6 · · · · · · · · 7 · · · · · · · · 8 · · · · · · · · 9 · · · · · · · 1 0

Not desperate at all.   I really want this to work.   It feels like my life depends on it.

How have you blamed yourself for the failure of a diet or fitness plan?

Work It Out

Read and write down your observations from the following verses. If your life has ever felt like one long attempt to stick to a diet, what do these verses speak to you?

John 6:35

Psalm 107:9

Psalm 16:11

1 Corinthians 10:31

Luke 12:23

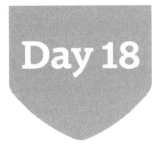

Day 18

It Was Never about the Food

The unstable faith of dieting

> Their loyalty is divided between God and the world, and they are unstable in everything they do.
>
> *James 1:8 NLT*

In my late twenties, I followed a popular diet plan where you "enjoyed" two shakes and a packaged snack bar each day and then ate a balanced dinner. I wanted to lose weight before an upcoming vacation, so, like a gambler betting it all on black, I jumped into this new plan with gusto.

Until the day I forgot to take my snack bar to work. I snuck out to the drugstore and discovered a new flavor. Ravenous, I ripped open that bar in the parking lot. Its crunchy, peanut-buttery goodness enraptured my starving body. Then it hit me. It tasted just like a Butterfinger. *How could that be?* I went back in and bought more of my diet bars and several Butterfingers so I could conduct a blind taste test among my office mates.

Soon I'd made two discoveries. First, according to the label, my diet bar and the Butterfinger were nearly nutritionally identical. The diet bar was smaller, so it had fewer calories and less sugar, and it was fortified with vitamins that the Butterfinger lacked. But the actual ingredients list was almost interchangeable and ordered similarly.

Second, my coworkers could not tell the difference between the diet bar and the Butterfinger. While I believed I was making nutritionally excellent choices for my health by following this program, these "smarter" snacks were just shrunken candy bars. *The truth hurts.*

What hurt even more was that those diet bars cost four times as much as the candy bars. I could have saved hundreds of dollars by simply taking a vitamin and eating half a Butterfinger at the appointed snack time.

I never followed that program again. But that doesn't mean I didn't find another one that boasted even more superior health consciousness and better results, of course.

And this proves the depth of my faith in diets. **Instead of questioning the legitimacy of the diets, I determined the real problem was me.**

Unstable Faith

Faith in so-called "right" eating always lets us down. **There's no absolute truth in the dieting world. The rules always change.** In college, you couldn't have paid me to eat an avocado. *Do you know how much fat is in one of those?* Fat-free bagels dominated my mealtimes.

By the time I hit thirty, I ordered guacamole at every Mexican restaurant but schemed ways to eat it without the carbohydrate-laden chips. *Are baby carrots on the menu?* I tried being a vegetarian in my twenties because I worried about eating all that protein. But by age forty, I sustained myself with protein bars, almonds, and hamburgers without the bun.

Argue what you wish about what the "best" foods are for your body now, but one thing I know for certain: **Fickle food trends haven't made any of us healthier.**

Tracy Brown, a non-diet dietitian friend, appeared on my podcast to explain how the cycling of "acceptable foods" versus "bad-for-you foods" shouldn't surprise us. There are only three macronutrients: carbohydrates, fat, and protein. Each one gets a turn as king of the nutrient hill, while another gets booted to the naughty list. Tracy explained how when you suppress the intake of one macronutrient for an extended time, your body will eventually crave that nutrient more than any others. So by the time your body is weary of low-carb living, don't worry—diet culture will label bread safe again.

Anyone else feeling jerked around? Like with a bad boyfriend—it's hard to break up with diet culture. *What if everyone gets the body of their dreams and I'm left behind?* Meanwhile, our nutrition suffers as we follow fads. Our quest for a thinner body can often lead to muscle loss, hormonal imbalances, bone density issues, infertility, blood sugar regulation issues, frequently feeling cold, and thyroid and adrenal problems.[1] **If your food plan makes you lose your hair, your period, or your sex drive, it's not improving your health.** Undereating, no matter what you weigh, can increase your heart rate and decrease your ability to fight infections.[2]

Our decisions to follow diets aren't flippant. They are deeply spiritual, emotional, and physical. Food restriction or an eat/binge/eat cycle may be born from trauma, rejection, or neglect in our past. We long for much more than body change, so we're willing to do whatever it takes, hoping the plan will take the pain away. Strong emotions connect to our habits with food and eating.

They Loved Food Rules

In 2012, Intermittent Fasting (IF) hit the dieting scene, and it seemed like the answer to everyone's prayer. Finally, food freedom! IF isn't about *what* you eat, but *when*. Today, I'm watching IF fade out of style like wall-to-wall shag carpet. New data show that eating windows don't really matter to weight loss or health. Dr. Ethan Weiss, lead researcher, "Used to be a true believer in time-restricted eating and said that for seven years he had eaten only between noon and 8 p.m." Further research failed to demonstrate any benefits to this approach. Weiss confessed, "I was a devotee. . . . This was a hard thing to accept."[3] *Sigh. But will breakfast ever earn back its title as the most important meal of the day? Stay tuned . . .*

What if all these rules we create around our food keep us from pursuing the One who knows our bodies better than any influencer? Concepts espoused by diet culture come from people, not Scripture. Even "truth" backed by the latest medical research is subject to change. We must not cling too tightly to any of the wisdom offered by this world. *Remember when doctors thought bloodletting*

1. Jennifer L. Gaudiani, *Sick Enough: A Guide to the Medical Complications of Eating Disorders* (New York: Routledge, 2019).

2. Micah Abraham, "Anxiety and Appetite Problems," Calm Clinic, October 10, 2020, https://www.calmclinic.com/anxiety/symptoms/appetite-problems.

3. Gina Kolata, "Scientists Find No Benefit to Time-Restricted Eating," *The New York Times*, April 20, 2022, https://www.nytimes.com/2022/04/20/health/time-restricted-diets.html.

was a solid idea? Only God's capital-T Truth is eternal. Our beliefs around food and the body must always be held up against his truth.

In Mark 7:6–8, Jesus calls the Pharisees out for honoring God with their lips but teaching the commandments of men as doctrines. Do we also confuse food rules and wisdom from internet health gurus with God's absolute truth?

Read Mark 7:6–8. What do you think?

Remember those Pharisees? They took the ten rules of the Old Testament and turned them into more than six hundred. They had rules for following their rules. Sounds a little like diet culture, right? They wanted to be saved by their own efforts. Jesus said, "Follow me." They responded, "No thanks, we'll follow the rules."

Though the Pharisees missed it, Jesus frees us from the curse of the law. He invites us into the life of grace. Yes. We should apply wisdom to the way we feed and treat our bodies. But let's not ignore the opportunity to invite God, the one who made our bodies, in to help us make choices that honor his standards, not diet culture's ever-changing rules. Unlike putting faith in a diet, only faith placed in him will never disappoint.

Read 1 Corinthians 6:19. Then read all of 1 Corinthians 6. What additional observations can you make now that you have a greater context for this Scripture verse?

Is this verse a mandate for Christians to follow culture's food rules or maintain a culturally popular size or weight?

Diet Culture Food Rules Versus God's Food Rules

Read the verses in this chart to compare what is true about God's rules versus diet culture's food rules.

Culture Says	God Says
Certain foods are deemed clean or unclean.	Romans 14:20
Some foods are dangerous. Resist sin by avoiding certain foods.	Matthew 15:11
Resist certain foods to stay pure.	Ecclesiastes 9:7
Espouse that this plan is the "most healthy" way to eat.	Romans 14:2–4

Work It Out

Write down any rules you hold around food or eating. Where did these rules originate? Are they from your doctor? Your parents? A social media influencer?

Rules	Origination
Example: No food after 8 p.m.	Dieting article in magazine
Only eat carbs with protein	Fitness influencer on YouTube

Act

Not all rules are bad, but you may find that many are unhelpful and originate from an unknown or unqualified source. Choose one of these rules and break it this week. Pick an easy one and write down what happens when you break it. Did you feel like you had done something wrong? If so, how? How does your obligation to follow this rule change when you understand that it's a rule of culture instead of a part of God's moral law?

If this feels too hard, consider reaching out to a professional from the resource list in the back of this book.

Day 19

Get Thin Quick

What your body does on a diet

> To promise not to do a thing is the surest way in the world to make a body want to go and do that very thing.
>
> *Mark Twain*

A *Daily Mail* survey found that by age forty-five, the average woman has been on sixty-one diets.[1] If pollsters called me to ask how many diets I've been on, I wouldn't be able to count them all! *Did they mean new diets or just the Monday mornings I mustered up the energy to return to the old one? Should I count those twenty-two hours I was vegan?* Good thing they never rang. I would've muddied their data!

Theoretically, I like diets. They give me a sense of control. If I just follow the rules, I get the outcomes I desire. You do what the diet says is right. You get what you deserve. Perfect for those of us with a strong sense of justice.

Until you don't. Then you feel like a failure. *What's wrong?* You thought you were doing well. *Except for that one night.* The night the chips got you. *But it was just a few. Surely a couple handfuls of chips can't ruin two weeks' worth of dieting?* Your brain is riddled with perceived failure. *Might as well give up!*

Diet. Cheat. Repeat. This cycle isn't healthy for anyone—physically or mentally. If you really want to feel like a loser, just keep failing at the same unrealistic thing and blaming yourself for it. (This really helps you feel better about your

---

1. Daily Mail Reporter, "Women Have Tried 61 Diets by the Age of 45 in the Constant Battle to Stay Slim," *Daily Mail*, March 20, 2012, https://www.dailymail.co.uk/health/article-2117445/Women-tried-61-diets-age-45 -constant-battle-stay-slim.html.

body too. *Ugh! Not so much.*) That's what happens in the diet cycle. Yet somehow, we blame ourselves instead of the plans.

The Pathway to Eating Disorders

Nearly every eating disorder starts with a plan that restricts amounts or types of food. Behind opioid addictions, eating disorders are the second leading cause of mental illness–related deaths.[2] Though not everyone who diets has an eating disorder, everyone who engages in restrictive behaviors begins to develop disordered eating behaviors.[3]

Disordered Eating Behaviors

According to eatright.org, a resource of the Academy of Nutrition and Dietetics, *disordered eating* describes a wide range of behaviors that don't always merit a clinical diagnosis of an eating disorder. These can include but are not limited to:

- skipping meals
- feeling anxiety around eating specific foods and feeling guilt or shame about eating in general
- dieting frequently
- keeping strict routines, rules, or rituals around food (not merited by medical conditions)
- fixating on or having preoccupying thoughts about food, body image, and weight
- feeling a loss of control around food, including compulsive eating
- using exercise or food restriction to purge the body of "bad foods" or to make up for consuming certain foods.[1]

1. "What Is Disordered Eating?" October 26, 2018, https://www.eatright.org/health/health-conditions/eating-disorders/what-is-disordered-eating.

2. Eric Graber, "Eating Disorders Are on the Rise," *American Society for Nutrition*, February 22, 2021, https://nutrition.org/eating-disorders-are-on-the-rise/.
3. "Disordered Eating and Dieting," National Eating Disorders Collaboration, https://nedc.com.au/eating-disorders/eating-disorders-explained/disordered-eating-and-dieting/.

Thirty-five percent of "normal dieters" progress to pathological dieting. In other words, dieting becomes an addiction. Of those, one-fourth progress to full or partial-syndrome eating disorders.[4] **Restriction almost always leads to bingeing.**

Food restriction, calorie or macro restriction, avoiding certain foods because you're afraid they'll make you fat—all of these habits damage our bodies in the long run. When we lose weight through restriction, our bodies no longer feel safe. Your starving body doesn't know that you have a pantry full of food that's not on your plan. It only knows it's hungry and not being fed.

So like a ship that's about to sink, it may start tossing weight overboard. We celebrate this like a victory, but in truth, our body signals that something is wrong. To adapt, it may even shut off all unnecessary systems—reproduction being one of the first. (I lost my period for nine months during college. I thought it was just stress, but it was my body in distress!)[5]

What's That Buzz?

Then the buzz comes. I always loved the high after the first week of a new diet. I attributed it to how great the plan must be working. The adrenaline it stirred motivated me to keep going. I remember thinking, *I never want this feeling to end!*

But in an interview with accomplished eating disorder expert Amy Carlson, she exposed something startling. **The buzz that comes after the first week of a restrictive diet isn't a sign of success. It's your body shifting into hyperdrive to protect you from experiencing the pain of starvation.** You may feel like you're high on willpower, but your body is shouting, "Being without adequate food hurts! But don't worry, I'll protect you from feeling it so you can keep functioning!" In more primitive times, this extra adrenaline boost provided the calorie-free energy needed to go hunt or gather food to stay alive.

The serial dieter can't stop, because every time she goes off a diet, her body recovers by adding weight.[6] Depending on your genetics, trauma history, and

4. Catherine M. Shisslak, Marjorie Crago, and Linda S. Estes, "The Spectrum of Eating Disturbances," *International Journal of Eating Disorders* 18, no. 3 (November 1995): 209–19, https://onlinelibrary.wiley.com/doi /10.1002/1098-108X(199511)18:3%3C209::AID-EAT2260180303%3E3.0.CO;2-E.

5. This is related to a medical condition called hypothalamic amenorrhea.

6. "Set Point Theory" in "Getting Educated about Eating Disorders," Centre for Clinical Interventions, January 25, 2018, https://www.cci.health.wa.gov.au/~/media/CCI/Consumer-Modules/Break-Free-From-ED/Break-Free -From-ED---15---Getting-Educated-About-Eating-Disorders-Education-Pack.pdf.

dieting/bingeing/restricting/eating habits history, your body may add a lot or just a little.

Though we may groan in frustration, we should all stop and thank our bodies for doing this. The body is smart enough to know that if it faced famine once, it could face famine again. So it'll be better prepared next time and keep a few more pounds, just in case. **Your body's job is to keep you alive.**

Starvation and Dieting

A strange thing happened to me when I stopped dieting. I lost interest in the Food Network and I stopped Pinning dessert recipes. I didn't think about food as often. *What will I have for lunch?* no longer monopolized my morning thoughts.

In the 1940s, a team of researchers at the University of Minnesota studied the effects of starvation. The purpose of the study was to inform aid for war-torn countries facing food scarcity, so the War Department allowed men who were fit for military service (but consciously objecting) to participate as a form of public service.

These young men were psychologically and physically pictures of health. They underwent extensive testing and were deemed a happy, well-adjusted, and disciplined group. During the first few months, they were allowed to eat normally, and researchers noted no change in behavior or health.[7]

But as the experiment went on, their calories were cut in half, and crazy things happened. Hunger made the men obsessed. They fantasized about food, talked about food, and started reading cookbooks. Some rummaged through the trash or stole forbidden treats. The men grew irritable, depressed, and apathetic. They lost strength and stamina and felt fatigued. **Even after a five-month refeeding process, the men still ate more than they had before starvation.** Plus, afterward, they reported feeling hungrier, engaging in binge eating and purging behaviors, and developing body image issues.[8]

I won't tell you how many daily calories they were allowed during starvation, as calorie counts can be very triggering for those with eating disorders. But the number matches one I've repeatedly seen advertised as "ideal for weight loss."

---

7. David Baker and Natacha Keramidas, "The Psychology of Hunger," American Psychological Association, *Monitor on Psychology* 44, no. 9 (October 2013): 66, https://www.apa.org/monitor/2013/10/hunger.

8. Chantal Gil, "The Starvation Experiment," Duke Health, Center for Eating Disorders, https://eatingdisorders .dukehealth.org/education/resources/starvation-experiment.

Yet, as this research reminds us, starving our bodies only causes harm. Calorie restriction always has consequences.

Body by Sumo

Most women with body image issues aren't hoping to look more like a sumo wrestler. But it's ironic that many dieting principles we use to "get fit" are used by these athletes to maintain their hearty size and shape. Sumo wrestlers skip breakfast, exercise on an empty stomach, take a nap after meals, and only eat twice a day. They work out six days a week for hours each day. They do consume a lot of calories, but they eat lots of vegetables, rice, and high-protein foods. **Here's the real kicker: While diet culture would tell you that anyone who weighs upwards of three hundred pounds must be unhealthy, it's not true for sumo wrestlers.** They keep their weight within a consistent range and are metabolically healthy, with low cholesterol, and low risk for heart disease or stroke.[9]

It's important to note that we can't judge health by observing body size. **You can be healthy and not wear a single-digit size.** Likewise, it's also possible to wear smaller clothes sizes but struggle physically, emotionally, and mentally with food and your health. Despite what diet culture teaches, body size is not the ultimate symbol of how healthy you are.[10]

Work It Out

How has the information in the last few chapters changed or impacted your perspective on food and diet? Write down your top three takeaways.

1.

2.

3.

9. William, "What Is a Sumo Wrestlers Diet?" Master Fighting, https://masterfighting.com/what-is-a-sumo-wrestlers-diet/.

10. Linda Bacon and Lucy Aphramor, "Weight Science: Evaluating the Evidence for a Paradigm Shift," National Library of Medicine, *Nutrition Journal* 10, no. 9 (January 2011), https://www.ncbi.nlm.nih.gov/pmc/articles/PMC3041737/.

Act

Diets are about restriction, but it's what we *add* to our life that often leads to better health. There are many things you can do for your body to help you feel good. **Mark two of the sixteen ideas below you could incorporate into your routine this month.**

Things You Can Do to Improve Your Health Without Following a Diet

- Add one additional serving of vegetables daily.
- Add two extra glasses of water a day.
- Make time to sit and eat breakfast.
- Add a ten-minute walk to your midday or lunchtime routine.
- Add a midmorning snack of berries, nuts, or yogurt.
- Add a prayer before each meal, thanking God for the gift of food and your body.
- Add one full minute of deep breathing before each meal.
- Choose to eat according to your body's hunger signals, not the clock.
- Take the time to prepare a favorite food at home you'd usually order out.
- Sit and enjoy a meal without your phone, work, or other media distractions.
- Eat a midafternoon snack to regulate blood sugar.
- Invite a friend to eat a meal with you.
- Take time to really taste your food, naming in your head the flavors or textures you notice.
- Find a type of movement you enjoy and write it on your schedule so you can do it.
- Sit in the sunshine for ten minutes to soak in the vitamin D.
- Take a bath to de-stress at the end of hard days.
- Consult an eating disorder therapist if you feel unsettled around food.

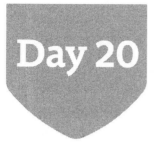

I've Never Confused Carrots for Chocolate

Nourishing our bodies

> It feels like we're in a war with food. But what if it's just a game of tug-of-war where no one is holding the other side of the rope?
>
> *Amy Carlson, MS, RD, LD*

It's 4 p.m. and I just had a cup of decaf and a donut because I'm trying to be healthier. *No, that wasn't sarcasm.*

It was my son's fifteenth birthday. If you've had a teenager, you may understand how the "let's celebrate by taking a treat to school" idea was met with less than giddy enthusiasm. But we homeschool. So for the good of his whole co-op class, I talked him into allowing me to purchase a dozen donuts for the seven of them.

You did the math already, didn't you? Seven people, twelve donuts. That leaves five unaccounted for. No worries, I have three other children. They each grabbed one. Two donuts remained.

I taught all afternoon with that pink donut box in my peripheral vision. Exhausted at the end of the day, I only wanted to go home and savor that donut-y goodness with a hot cup of coffee. So, I did it. I ate the donut.

The "old me" would have obsessed and talked herself out of it. She would have eaten a protein bar, a spoonful of peanut butter, and some fruit—while still wishing she had the donut. She would've overeaten at dinner because she denied her body what it craved. By 7 p.m., she'd have gone completely off the rails and started eating chocolate chips by the handful.

Then, after hours of donut fixation, she would've ripped off a piece of its soft, cakey goodness. Three minutes later, she'd return for another little piece. And she would have repeated this pattern until, you guessed it, she ate the whole donut. And maybe the second!

Eating what I want feels far from natural to me. I fight the "I shouldn't be free around food" belief system. Thoughts flood: *I didn't do anything to "earn" it. The holidays are coming; I'll probably overdo it then, so I should save up my calories.* Can you relate?

But I put my brain on silent and savored that delicious donut. And I felt satisfied. I didn't feel the need to rummage for more treats. In fact, I stared at the remaining donut and wasn't even tempted.

A healthy relationship with food isn't about knowing the nutritional value and calorie content of every morsel that enters your mouth. Instead, it's about having food in its proper place and learning that it's okay to crave and okay to satisfy your hunger cravings.

It's okay to crave? Haven't we been taught, like good soldiers in the diet culture army, that cravings are the enemy? *Christian women—you better only crave Jesus!* they shouted. Aim. Fire. Kill the cravings before they kill your results at the weigh-in. *You want crunch?* Substitute carrots for chips. *Do you want something sweet?* Remember those juicy oranges are just as delicious as chocolate.

But they aren't. Chips aren't carrots. Oranges aren't chocolate. Sometimes my body craves hearty vegetables or flavorful fruits. But my mouth refuses to be fooled into believing that nonfat yogurt tastes like sour cream. I can "win" the battle against my cravings for an hour, a few days, or weeks. But when my willpower runs out, I won't just have a couple chips. I'll eat the whole bag. *Children, hide your candy. Mommy is off her diet!*

No one is saying that donuts, chips, and chocolate should be staples of every meal. I'm not claiming they're nutritionally superior to cauliflower and almonds. But our bodies can be trusted to tell us what we need. After spending a lifetime following everyone else's advice, it takes time to listen to our bodies talk. **Food is just food.** Thinking about it doesn't have to consume our lives. Crazy thing, though: **Eating cures food fixation like nothing else can. When I stopped categorizing the foods I love as "bad," I stopped daydreaming about them.**

What about Self-Control?

Biblical self-control shouldn't be confused with food restriction. In fact, there's no reason to believe that denying our body the calories or nutrients it needs exemplifies the fruit of the Spirit. Self-control, according to Scripture, is about killing our sin nature, not letting our flesh (our old self and its desires) rule us. With self-control, we have boundaries in place that help us live more holy and righteous lives for Jesus, not for any selfish ambition of our own (like getting a "better" body). **Lest there be any confusion, eating isn't a sin. Neither is there a verse in the Bible that says you should never eat foods you enjoy.** Instead, eating is the best way to "take care of your temple" and be a good steward of it. God created us to eat.

Trying Not to Eat

It's still tempting to believe the concept that I can get smaller by skipping meals or restricting portions. But I never knew I had an eating disorder, because I wasn't thin "enough" to be in that category. "Trying not to eat" was my life's motto. Now I understand I likely had some atypical form of anorexia. I work with women every single week who, similarly, would've never believed they had an eating disorder. Yet thoughts and fears over food and weight consume their thoughts daily. This may be normative, but that doesn't make it healthy.

With an ever-growing list of food rules guiding me, I gradually learned to shut down the signals my body was created to give me in the arena of nourishment. Instead of understanding that my brain needs glucose to think, I believed my sugar craving was a sign of weakness. **Instead of understanding that my nonstop eating in the late afternoon was because I had starved myself all day long, I labeled myself an emotional eater who needed better restraint.** Controlling my body was my duty. I never paused to recognize that God created my body to run on food. Messages from diet culture that told me not to eat didn't align with God's truth. Hunger, cravings, and other signals from my body need to be nurtured, not ignored in the name of health. Our bodies were designed to communicate with us, but dieting teaches us to turn those notifications off.

How would you describe your relationship with food today?

Intuitive Eating

I've adopted a more natural way to eat that also allows us to appreciate the way God designed our bodies. It's called *intuitive eating*, but it's not as intuitive as it sounds. It's not as simple as just eating what you want, when you want—at least not for most of us who have been on a diet (or twelve). Changing how you think and feel around food is a complex process. There's a necessary breaking up with a restriction and a food morality mindset. **Intuitive eating without cognizant separation from the messages of diet culture just becomes an off-the-wagon binge.**

If food feels like too dangerous a topic, take it slow. How you eat may be filled with sacred rituals developed because you believe they help you control your body size or health. Some of what you're doing may be helpful. For example, a plan that requires you to eat every few hours may have instilled a habit of regular fueling that keeps your blood sugar stable. Likewise, there's wisdom in good nutrition. There are certain foods that make us feel good, while others may make us feel fuzzy or lethargic. Food allergies/intolerances are real. Genetic differences mean that not every food is healthy for every body. **Finding what nourishes you requires tuning in to your individual body and tuning out what's trending.**

Until you feel safe in your body—no matter what size, shape, or appearance it has—you will not feel free to make changes with the way you relate to food. If you're not ready to go there yet, come back to this chapter.

Created to Eat

While teaching a class on English grammar, I wrote the sentence "Eating is healthy" on the whiteboard to illustrate a gerund. Within seconds, several of my eleven- and twelve-year-old students clamored to change it. They wanted it rewritten as "Eating certain foods is healthy." They fought back as if the sentence made an outlandish claim. This fundamental premise that eating *is* good for our bodies and that eating is how we were created to survive had already been skewed in their brains. (*Thank you, diet culture.*)

Throughout the Bible, Jesus uses nourishment to illustrate what he offers us because he expects us to understand this from our experiences with food! Eating, drinking, refreshment, filling, stabilizing, healing, energizing—Scripture's illustrations should be relatable because God created us to feel physical hunger, and he gave us food to satisfy it. He designed our bodies to provide that warm surge of rest that comes when your belly is full and happy.

Yet our relationship with food has become so distorted and disordered that we may have convinced ourselves that nourishment is wrong. But this couldn't be further from the truth. Remember, God will throw us a magnificent heavenly feast—the Marriage Supper of the Lamb (Revelation 19:6–9).

Eating won't be necessary for our new, heavenly bodies to function. We won't be hungry (Revelation 7:16). Yet God wants us to celebrate him with food! *Can someone please explain that to those who've perpetuated the food fearmongering?* God wants us to enjoy food!

Yes, God created every system of our body to be sustained by nutrients. Our brain runs on carbohydrates, and our cells are built by protein. We store fats for energy, but they also insulate us and protect our vital organs. Without enough food, we harm our bodies. Jesus calls himself the Bread of Life because he wants to fill and satisfy us even more than a warm loaf of sourdough does.

Taste and See

There's wisdom in nourishing our bodies well, but ever-changing food rules bind us to a system of false beliefs touting that we can control our bodies if we just follow specific rules. Over a lifetime, we may keep adding new rules until there's not much left that's "legal." This is bondage. I remember walking into the kitchen many times, ravenous but unable to find something to eat, while ignoring a bowl full of apples and bananas because of my fear of carbs. If you're hungry and have food available but cannot eat because of a rule, you may be enslaved to a principle that isn't biblical.

It's not that structure around food is wrong. Instead, we must consider whose rules dictate that structure. Are you free to choose foods you enjoy that energize your body? Or do you feel forced to follow the food trends of the day?

Scripture tells us to "taste and see that the LORD is good" (Psalm 34:8). Have food rules and dieting zapped all the joy out of your ability to taste and see that food is good? Why would God even use the analogy of taste if he didn't want us to enjoy food as an illustration of the way we should enjoy him?

Work It Out

Nourishment is what is good and necessary for our growth, health, and condition. Scripture talks about ways that we nourish our bodies both physically and spiritually. Look up these verses on nourishment and jot down your thoughts beside each one.

The Fab Four of Nourishment

Psalm 34:8

Proverbs 3:8

John 4:32–34

Acts 9:19

What other words do you observe in Scripture that are used to describe our spiritual nourishment?

How does your approach or attitude toward food change after observing the language God uses around food and nourishment?

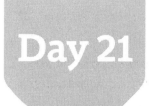

Good Foods/Bad Foods

What diet culture teaches about satisfaction

> Blessed are those who hunger and thirst for righteousness, for they shall be satisfied.
>
> *Matthew 5:6 ESV*

I'm a clearance shopper. I never shop from the front of the store; I stick to the 75 percent off racks in the back. Though I may tell you I'm frugal, the truth is, it's hard for me to buy nice things for myself. I wrestle to believe that I deserve what I really want.

So I settle. Instead of choosing what I love, spending a little more, and being satisfied with my purchases, I keep buying what's leftover and marked down. My habits have led to a closet filled with items that lack my luster. There's a row of ten tops that I paid less than twelve dollars each for, but I don't really love any of them. Would it have been better for me to buy the one beautiful sixty-dollar blouse than the ten cheap ones that I won't wear next year? Probably. But my issue isn't economic. **I'm uncomfortable with satisfaction. This trickles into my body image and food issues too.**

I've never been satisfied with my body. That number in the size tag I was sure would make me content, didn't. It's difficult to say "God made my body good" when body dysmorphia[1] and eating disorders fog your goggles.

---

1. Body dysmorphic disorder (BDD) is a mental health condition where you can't stop thinking about your body, your appearance, or your size. Body frustration affects your ability to live life normally. There are many varied symptoms of BDD that can be diagnosed by a mental health professional.

Likewise, I spent many decades feeling like it was wrong to derive pleasure from food. Meals didn't have to be gross, but there was a certain piety to forking down dry arugula instead of savoring salad dressing.

Even the words we use to describe delicious foods imply that enjoying food is somehow evil. We call molten lava cake "sinfully" delicious, while fat-free, sugar-free sandwich cookies are labeled "guilt-free." Diet culture has conditioned us to think about food in black-and-white terms. Good foods. Bad foods. You're indulgent if you like it, holy if you abstain.

Eat the toast without the jelly to save calories. Better yet, skip the toast altogether. Save more. We follow these mottos for "healthier" living, but is this really what's healthiest for our bodies?

Eating is more than fueling. It's an experience, a celebration of life. **When we believe diet culture's lie that delicious food is to be feared, we take a good gift of God and trample it.** God didn't have to create sweet pineapples or strawberries. He could have chosen to sustain our bodies with daily manna, as he did for the Israelites. But instead, he gave us tastebuds to distinguish a wide variety of flavors and textures. Satisfaction is about enjoying what we eat.

It's about the jelly, the flavored creamer, the butter, and the whipped topping too. I'm not arguing that these condiments are the nutritional equivalent of kale, but they add joy and delight to eating. Why would God have led his people to the promised land of "milk and honey" if he wanted their lives to be flavor-free? He knew that a little bit of richness and sweetness would bring delight. When Jesus turned water into wine, the crowd at the wedding feast didn't ask if it was low sugar. Instead, they remarked that the wedding host had saved the best wine for last. In other words, it was enjoyable (John 2:2–11)!

Every dieter knows that weeks of bland food can turn a cheery disposition sour. I picture God watching us always refuse dessert and questioning *Why?* Yes, there are times we purposefully deny ourselves for the cause of Christ, but that's different from constantly denying ourselves satisfying food for the cause of a "better looking" body.

If the practice of denial makes it more difficult for me to love others well, it conflicts with one of my main missions for life. When I restricted foods that taste good, it made me grumpy and affected my relationships. I'm not exaggerating when I say that when I stopped restricting and started eating foods I enjoy, my marriage improved.

When eating food consistently lacks satisfaction, willpower fades. Our bodies refuse to stay unsatisfied forever. There's a spiritual lesson to be learned here too. Throughout Scripture, we're encouraged to be satisfied in Jesus. If we make our relationship with Jesus black coffee and plain toast, there's not much to love. It's duty and obligation, not joy. God loves to delight his children with good gifts. Food is one of them.

Dissatisfaction gets us into trouble in many arenas. Few who are satisfied in their marriage consider cheating on their spouse. If you're satisfied with your finances, you're not tempted to fudge the truth on your taxes or overwork to the detriment of family and friendships. Satisfaction yields rest. Satisfaction yields peace. **Dissatisfaction may share a bunk with the root of all evil.**

Likewise, a wrestling match to find satisfaction in Jesus and not jelly donuts presents a false dichotomy. Sure, I can't love donuts *more* than Jesus. **But I'm hard-pressed to find a verse that tells me enjoying food is wrong.** Scripture uses satisfaction with food as a frequent metaphor for finding satisfaction in the Lord. God never tells us to mute our cravings to get (or stay) skinny. He only instructs us to find our *greatest* satisfaction in him.

Healthy Satisfaction

Though diet culture has convinced us that we'll always feel better choosing rice cakes over cupcakes, eating without satisfaction is actually *less* healthy for your body. A 2012 study showed that having a salad with lower-fat dressing instead of its full-fat counterpart limited the absorption of the nutrients—the carotenoids—found in the vegetables![2]

Digestion begins in the brain. How you think about your food actually impacts how well you digest it. If you are stressing as you eat it, your nutrient absorption level changes.[3] A 2011 study aptly called "Mind over Milkshakes" showed that people who believed they were making a good choice for their body

---

2. Purdue University, "Study: No-Fat, Low-Fat Dressings Don't Get Most Nutrients out of Salads," ScienceDaily, June 19, 2012, https://www.sciencedaily.com/releases/2012/06/120619230234.htm.
3. American Psychological Association, "Stress Effects on the Body," American Psychological Association, November 1, 2018, https://www.apa.org/topics/stress/body.

by drinking a milkshake labeled "healthy" triggered a stable ghrelin response compared to those who were told they were drinking something "bad" and who experienced a steeper decline in ghrelin. Ghrelin, the hormone responsible for signaling you are satisfied, allowed the "health drink" group to feel full and stop drinking their milkshake earlier than the indulgent group (most of whom emptied their glasses).[4] Stressing over whether or not you "should" eat a certain food puts the body in a fight or flight response. As my friend Erin Kerry, integrative nutrition coach, says, "A body that's stressed will not digest."

It's no wonder we're stressed out around food. **Diet culture has taught us we can't be trusted to make the right choices for our bodies** without a plan to follow. Perhaps parents, partners, or others have told us we don't manage our food choices well. But God is a good Father. He does not sit in heaven counting your calories. **God trusts you around food.** He's numbered the hairs on your head, not the macros on your plate. You are precious to him.

Work It Out

The Sweet Sixteen of Satisfaction

Satisfaction isn't wrong—in fact, Scripture talks about being satisfied in Christ more than sixteen times. Many of these illustrations include food.

Look up some or all of these verses and write down your responses. What do you observe about God's perspective on satisfaction?	
Psalm 107:9	**Psalm 145:16**
Psalm 63:5	**Psalm 132:15**
Proverbs 13:25	**Ecclesiastes 3:13**

4. A. J. Crum, W. R. Corbin, K. D. Brownell, and P. Salovey, "Mind over Milkshakes: Mindsets, Not Just Nutrients, Determine Ghrelin Response," *Health Psychology* 30, no. 4 (July 2011): 424–9, https://pubmed.ncbi.nlm.nih.gov/21574706/.

Psalm 22:26	Psalm 36:8
Ecclesiastes 5:18	Psalm 34:10
Joel 2:25–26	Isaiah 55:1–2
Luke 6:21	1 Timothy 6:17–19
Matthew 5:6	Psalm 147:14

Act

Does it feel scary to think about eating food that satisfies you? If so, in what way?

Are there other areas of your life where you avoid satisfaction?

Is it easy or hard for you to believe that being satisfied by food is a healthy and natural physical response created in our bodies by the God who gave us tastebuds?

Write your thoughts and feelings about God's view of satisfaction below. Can you believe that satisfaction is okay?

Transform Your Thinking

Day 22

Renewing Your Thought Life

Separating condemnation from conviction

> The first thing you lose on a diet is your sense of humor.
>
> *Anonymous*

In the C. S. Lewis book *The Screwtape Letters*, we read stories of scheming demons. But I realized there's no need for the enemy to spend a lot of thought and time trying to take *me* out. All he needs is a box of Thin Mints.

Allow me to explain. Girl Scout cookie season always falls toward the beginning of a new year. You know, that time of year when you're still trying to keep the resolutions you've made about eating healthier? That sweet girl in her cute green uniform calls out from a cookie-laden table outside the grocery store, "Do you want to buy some Thin Mints?" *Well, of course I do, precious!*

But what happens next is as predictable as spam in my inbox. I call it *promise-busting*. You see, by the time I've handed that little girl a twenty-dollar bill, I've already broken a vow I made to myself last December while washing those Christmas cookie tins for storage. I swore, "No more cookies for me. I'm done."

It was a ridiculous vow, no doubt. But by filling my pantry with a rainbow of Girl Scout cookie boxes, I flirt with the very food I swore off just six weeks ago. Now I have a decision to make. *To cookie, or not to cookie? That is the question.*

The two lawyers in my head begin negotiations. The cookie defense team explains how Girl Scout cookies are a special treat—only available for one month a year. *How foolish I would be to miss that opportunity.* Meanwhile, the cookie prosecution reminds me that I'll never meet my body goals if I indulge. The judge sends them to mediation, and an agreement is reached. *I'll just eat a few. Today only. Just my favorites.* Can you relate?

Of course, there aren't *that* many cookies in those little boxes. So the next time I run into a desperate little Girl Scout, I buy more. And the process repeats, like that one episode of the TV show that you didn't really enjoy yet seems to be on every time you flip through the channels.

What's Happening in Our Heads?

We've talked about the ways we've been lied to by diet culture and marketers, but let's take a closer look at what's happening in our heads. Yes, shame is part of it. Guilt hangs out there too. But as we get better at picking out the lies of the enemy, we must learn to distinguish condemnation from conviction.

Simply put, condemnation comes from the enemy, and conviction comes from the Holy Spirit. It's often difficult to tell them apart, and sometimes we can even convince ourselves that the enemy's condemnation is helpful. When you feel bad after eating a whole can of Pringles, it may seem deserved that condemnation would come and help you "shape up" your eating habits. That's the tricky thing about the enemy's lies: They always contain some element of truth. If the enemy tried to tell you that Pringles are a vegetable, you wouldn't fall for it. But by convincing you that you shouldn't eat tomorrow because you ate Pringles today—Satan becomes a weight loss accountability partner.

Wait, what?

For Jesus followers, condemnation is never from the Lord, so we never have to listen to it. In fact, Scripture tells us that there is no condemnation for those who are in Christ (Romans 8:1). We don't have to live as those who are condemned. We've been declared righteous and free.

Too many of us live condemned for our food choices—as if eating something culture labels "bad" is a scarlet letter. (Even though all those green diet powders and clean protein bars are processed too! *Oops!*) I can find nowhere in my Bible that says this is a Christian, healthy, or helpful way to live. **Instead, I read that Jesus doesn't condemn us for what we eat.** Can you believe he even spells this out for us? "It is not what goes into the mouth that defiles a person, but what comes out of the mouth; this defiles a person" (Matthew 15:11 ESV).

Look up Matthew 15:11. How does Jesus's bold statement about food compare with what is taught by diet culture?

Condemnation Versus Conviction

Condemnation accompanies shame and makes us feel like we should hide or run to an idol to save us. **If those voices in your head start scolding you or convincing you that there's something deeply wrong with you because you didn't say no to a Thin Mint, this is condemnation. It's not from God.**

Conviction, on the other hand, is the way the Holy Spirit gently leads us and guides us to right living. We can trust that if we lean not on our own understanding (Proverbs 3:5–6) and ask the Lord to guide us, he will help us. But his conviction won't lead to shame or unhealthy solutions. The Holy Spirit's role is to instruct you toward holiness, not in the rules of the keto plan. Praise God that he offers us grace as we learn to relate to food in healthier ways. His mercies are new every morning. Know that God is not the one replaying in your head what you ate yesterday or how "bad" your food choices were last weekend. This is the enemy.

Guilt and shame are never Jesus's answer to the ways we struggle. He provided a cure for our sin and shame on the cross. His answer is to confess the sin, return to him, and walk in the Spirit again, forgiven. If you rely on God to help you make decisions around food, you can trust that his gentle conviction will tell you when you've had enough. But the Holy Spirit won't call you "fatty" or remind you repeatedly that you finished the rest of the box after you said you'd only eat two.

Now, you may be waiting for me to bring up gluttony. *What if it's not condemnation, but the Holy Spirit convicting me of my sin of gluttony?* We'll explore gluttony more tomorrow.

So back to me and that green box of crunchy, chocolaty goodness. When I feel bad about eating the cookies, how can I tell whether or not that's conviction or condemnation? Is it the enemy shaming me? Or is it the Holy Spirit trying to gently show me that sugar won't really cure my stress? Here are some ways to tell.

Conviction Versus Condemnation

Conviction comes from the Holy Spirit to help us grow and to guide us in the way that is right. There's no condemnation for the one who is in Christ (Romans 8:1).

Conviction	Condemnation
Brings us to closer connection with God	Attempts to separate us from God
Protects us	Guilts us
Is hope-filled	Brings shame, depression, or anxiety
Is specific and targeted to lead us to repentance	Is hopeless: *"You'll never get better"*
	Is vague and generalizing: *"You are lazy"*
Sounds like:	*Sounds like:*
You've been turning to exercise instead of prayer; turn to me.	*Shame on you for overeating—again.*
You're stressed.	*You have no restraint.*
	You're a slob.
Come to me, I want to help. Ice cream can't fix this, but I can.	*Get your act together.*
	What is your problem?

Work It Out

What words of condemnation do you hear in your head around food, body, or exercise? Write them below.

How does the chart above help free you from the shame or frustration they cause?

Act

~~~~~~

Go back to your lies list you created on Day 4. Write your top three in the space below, and then write what you believe Jesus would say instead.

Lie 1:

Jesus's response:

Lie 2:

Jesus would say:

Lie 3:

Jesus tells me:

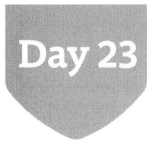

Day 23

Arrested for Gluttony

Legalism and the food police

> Laughter is brightest where food is best.
>
> *Irish Proverb*

Just seeing a police car makes me feel guilty. Aside from a small collection of speeding tickets, I don't have a history of trouble with the law, but the mere presence of a sedan with lights and a siren puts a pit in my stomach. I worry that I'm doing something wrong. *Did I break a driving rule I don't remember?*

The same sort of guilt and fear surfaced when I broke the laws of diet land. *Wow, did I hear those sirens blare!* The food police staked out in my pantry, close to where I hid the chocolate. One indulgence and they arrested me with shame. Their interrogations lasted for hours . . . sometimes days. *What did you eat? How will you pay for these crimes?* they taunted.

Separating shouts of the food police from whispers of the Holy Spirit further complicated the situation. I knew I'd gone off plan, but it felt like I'd broken God's rules too. Was God waiting for me to find more willpower around food? Were the food police sent by the Holy Spirit to help me? *Was this gluttony?*

What Is Gluttony?

While most would describe gluttony as eating too much food, there's not biblical evidence for this as the best definition. **Overeating and undereating are** normal parts of the human experience. Sometimes you don't even know you've eaten too much until it's too late. God doesn't play gotcha! Gluttony isn't what happens every Thanksgiving or when you're stressed after a long day at work. Like most of what Jesus confronts in the New Testament, gluttony is more about our hearts than the calories.

In the English Standard Version of the Bible, the word *glutton(s)* appears only six times, and four of those times it's paired with the word *drunkard*. The word *gluttonous* appears only once, also accompanying *drunkards*. There's an oft-cited verse in Proverbs 23:2 about putting a knife to your throat before eating too much of the king's rich food. But this verse is rightly interpreted as a caution against being swayed by the deceit of wealth and power, not as a warning against overeating.[1] In fact, some translations of verse Proverbs 23:8 clarify that you'll vomit up "the little you have eaten" (NIV). If eating just a little of this food makes one sick, how could this passage be about overeating? It saddens me that some have been fat-shamed by this passage out of context.

So who started the rumor that gluttony equals overeating? It was a fourth-century ascetic, gnostic monk. Considering monastic life, food may have been one of only a few possible vices for Evagrius Ponticus, who offered a food-centered definition of gluttony as one of the seven vices.[2] Some of his teachings were later adapted by Pope Gregory and woven into tenants of the Catholic faith. But Evagrius was later accused of heresy and mysticism. Gnostics separate body and spirit, and ascetics feel more spiritual when they deny the body everything. Consider the source. Note: It wasn't Jesus.

This history has influenced how we think about gluttony today. Yet in New Testament lists of sins (1 Corinthians 5:10–11; Galatians 5:19–21; and Ephesians 5:3–5, for example), drunkenness makes the list but gluttony does not. Neither is gluttony mentioned in the original Ten Commandments from the Old Testament. Of course, the Jewish people had many food rules, but Peter's vision in Acts 10 changed that paradigm. **The only eating-related sin in the New Testament is found in 1 Corinthians 11:27, taking the bread of communion unworthily.** The concept of gluttony has been co-opted by a twisting or

---

1. Kevin DeYoung, "But What about Gluttony!?!" The Gospel Coalition, April 24, 2014, https://www.thegospel coalition.org/blogs/kevin-deyoung/but-what-about-gluttony/.
2. DeYoung, "But What About Gluttony!?!"

misinterpretation of Scripture over the centuries. **Remember: Jesus was accused of being a glutton.** (See Matthew 11:19.) This likely had nothing to do with how much or what he ate. Instead, Jesus spent time with those who were far from God. The gluttons and the drunkards tried to party their way to better lives *until* they met Jesus.

Does this mean we can never sin in our relationship with food? Of course not. But to be clear, gluttony isn't about the quantity or nutritional value of the food we eat. It's about putting food in a role reserved for God. Gluttony focuses on self-satisfaction and self-indulgence; it's greedy and consumed with its own desires. The one who "lives to party" or elevates eating experiences that gratify the senses over living as Christ's disciple could be gluttonous. If you think of food as the most important thing in your life, it's worth pausing to evaluate. Overindulgence in food won't meet emotional and spiritual needs any more than restriction can make us righteous.

But that doesn't mean comfort eating equals gluttony. When Jesus's disciples were at a low point after his death and resurrection, what did the risen Jesus do? He made them breakfast (John 21:1–14). He was the Bread of Life, but he didn't ignore their physical needs. Being soothed through eating is a response we're born with. Is the infant who wants to keep nursing a glutton? *I don't think so.*

In *The Screwtape Letters*, C. S. Lewis delineates a type of gluttony few talk about—the gluttony of delicacy. **This form of gluttony connects more to keeping food rules than overeating.**[3] The experienced demon uncle explains that the only attention given to gluttony is the gluttony of excess, not the type of gluttony that prevents us from loving others well because we lack hospitality around food.

I've been guilty of this. "I couldn't possibly eat that. Do you know how many carbs it has?" *How did Lewis know to write about these secrets eighty years ago?* Afraid of what she'll be served, the one wrestling the gluttony of delicacy will turn down dinner invitations. Or her dietary preferences will be so hard to accommodate that she may stop receiving them. I've had many clients who avoid social situations because they can't control the menu.

---

3. C. S. Lewis, *The Screwtape Letters* (San Francisco: Harper Collins, 2001), 87.

This preoccupation with food or food avoidance may also be defined as gluttony. **Secret thoughts and obsessions with food, even if never exhibited in front of others, may be even more of a problem for us, spiritually, than the act of eating too much.** Choosing to honor food rules over the opportunity to fellowship may elevate food to a place in our hearts that is above what God asks of us.

How would you have defined gluttony?

Have you ever avoided a social situation or turned down an invitation because of uncertainty over what food would be served? Write about it here.

Overthinking Food

There's a distinction to be made when it comes to overthinking food. If you find yourself obsessing over food, it may be a physiological response to deprivation, not gluttony. Remember the University of Minnesota's starvation experiment? There's always a mental impact when the body is denied food. A hungry body will scheme to find nourishment.

Likewise, if you've starved your body all day long and you get home after work and find yourself eating nonstop until bedtime—know that this behavior isn't necessarily gluttonous either. Your body is doing what it was designed to do to keep you alive. If you're truly concerned that your eating habits cross the line into gluttony, seek out a professional from the link in the "Need More Help?" section in the back of this book. They can help you restore a healthy relationship with food.

But What about Overeating?

Is it possible to eat too much? *Of course.* Is it always a sin? There's no way to accurately extrapolate that from Scripture. Remember, the Jewish people had parties where they feasted for days! This misinterpretation of gluttony is likely rooted in legalism, the same religion that the Pharisees espoused. It keeps us counting and tracking to make sure we never go above an arbitrary amount of food we've set for ourselves. But even in that, the standard is hardly scientific. Who told you that was the right number of calories or macros for *your* body? *You've eaten too much as compared to whom?* Some days our bodies need more food because we're more active. Other days they need less. Without a metabolic testing system and a whole lot of scientific gear, the only way we can measure whether we're eating enough, too much, or too little is through listening to our bodies.

If you regularly eat to the point of feeling sick or feel like you can't stop eating once you start, you may have an eating disorder. Similarly, if you're not eating enough or using laxatives, purging, obsessing over food, over-exercising, or chewing food and spitting it out, seek professional help.

Note: There's no need to allow the food police or others to shame you into believing that a larger body symbolizes gluttony or that gluttony is the same as not following a diet. Neither claim is accurate. Atypical anorexia—anorexia without significantly low weight—comprises up to one-half of patients undergoing eating disorder treatment. Women and men with medium- and larger-sized bodies with significant amounts of "extra" weight can face the same life-threatening outcomes as those who are underweight.[4] **You cannot tell how much someone eats simply by looking at them.**

Work It Out

Read 1 Corinthians 6:12. How do you think this informs your relationship with food?

4. Kate Siber, "You Don't Look Anorexic," *The New York Times*, October 18, 2022, https://www.nytimes.com/2022/10/18/magazine/anorexia-obesity-eating-disorder.html.

Could thinking about food all day long be just as gluttonous as overeating? Write your thoughts here:

Do You Overexercise?

Movement is good, but overexercising can damage our bodies. We can be gluttonous in our approach to working out. Using exercise as a way to purge calories can be a sign of an eating disorder. See how many of these potential symptoms of overexercise are true for you. If you mark more than four, consider talking to a counselor or eating disorder specialist about ways you can have a healthier relationship with exercise:

- ☐ "No pain, no gain" is always my motto. I work till it hurts.
- ☐ If I feel like I've eaten too much, I always have to work out.
- ☐ I feel guilty if I skip a workout or take a rest day.
- ☐ I'm energized immediately after exercise but exhausted later.
- ☐ I crave sweets at night on days I work out.
- ☐ My muscles are regularly sore for more than four days after working out.
- ☐ I get sick a lot (decreased immune response).
- ☐ My resting heart rate is high.
- ☐ It's hard for me to skip a workout, even if I'm invited to do something fun.
- ☐ I never feel satisfied with the results of my workouts.
- ☐ Exercise is a way to "make up for" eating the "wrong" foods.

We'll cover what a healthy relationship with exercise looks like on Day 28.

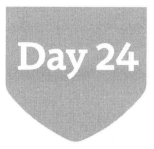

Day 24

Pimples, Wrinkles, and Fat

Fighting body fear

> Wrinkles will only go where the smiles have been.
>
> *Jimmy Buffet*

Aging is terrifying.

There, I said it. I should have more empathy for my teenagers and parents—but I'm too busy coping with aging's impact on my life. *What is this extra cushion around my waist and when did tweezing hairs become my new hobby?*

Gerascophobia—the fear of aging—is an actual condition. It's not those who can no longer fit all their candles on their birthday cake that struggle with it the most. It's women turning twenty-five who are panicked that they're halfway to fifty. I understand. Thirty once felt ancient to me too. It seems *old* is a relative word we use to define someone twenty years our senior.

But there's no reason to fear aging. God tells us that getting older is a gift. Gray hair is a crown and long life is a blessing (Proverbs 16:31; Psalm 91:16). *But it sure doesn't feel that way sometimes.*

So why do we stress? What we really fight is fear. Fear can wear many name tags—anxiety, control, shame, depression, or approval—but fear is the puppet master behind each of them. And fear is central to all our body image and comparison issues. In the past few years as I've been writing and speaking about body image, I've received many notes from women who've read my books on body image and comparison or listened to my "Compared to Who?" podcast. See if you can see the fear theme:

"I am haunted daily by the *fear* of becoming fat. This has been a lifelong struggle, and I desperately want to be free of the grip and *fear* of my body image."

"I have been a *slave* to the scale my entire life. It's the prominent fixture in my bathroom. Whatever it says *rules* my feelings for the day. I'm often *afraid* to step on it."

"People called me Casper the Friendly Ghost and asked if I was afraid of the sun. They didn't know how *self-conscious* I was of my pale skin. I was *afraid* I could never be beautiful because I couldn't tan."

Save Me, Please!

When we feel afraid, what is the first thing we do? We look for something to rescue us. *What can make me feel safe again?* These feelings turn us all into avid buyers of all the body transformation plans, supplements, creams, and potions. *If $29.95 a month can save me, I'm in!* **When fear is your uber driver, it'll take you wherever it wants to go.**

Circle any of these statements that relate to you.

I've been afraid that others won't think I'm pretty.

I've been afraid I'll be rejected for the way I look.

I've been afraid I'll never find a man.

I've been afraid my man will find someone who looks better than me and leave.

I've been afraid others won't accept me.

I've been afraid others will judge me for the way I look.

I've been afraid others will assume I'm unhealthy, uneducated, or lazy because of how I look.

I've been afraid I'm not attractive enough to do the things I want to do or accomplish my God-given dreams.

Deepest Fears

Fear is never from God. He tells us to trust him and not be afraid. He doesn't condemn us for our fear; rather, he offers a solution for it: faith in him.

A few years ago, I did a podcast on this topic, and as I prepared, I felt like God showed me an important distinction about fear as it relates to our body image. Though I distract myself from my fear with quests to improve myself, what if my biggest fear isn't whether or not I'm enough? **What if my real fear is whether God is enough?**

In what ways has fear as it relates to your body image impacted you? Think of ways it affected your thought life, how you dressed, what you ate, who you spent time with, etc., . . . and list them below.

Who Told Us Our Body Is the Enemy?

I recently received an email from a woman who found my podcast while she was in the waiting room to get Botox. She said she'd felt hesitant to ask God about getting it done, but she didn't know how else to fight the overwhelm of aging. Watching our bodies change in ways that are out of our control feels daunting. But why are we at war with our changing bodies?

We'd never tell a thirteen-year-old girl there's something wrong with her because her hips are spreading. **Similarly, there is nothing wrong with you if you're turning thirty, forty, fifty, or older, and your body is changing too.** During our twenties or thirties, we may notice little lines on our faces or gray hairs at our roots. As we reach our forties and beyond, our body shape may continue to shift or spread. But why would any of these changes be less culturally acceptable when we hit the midlife "pause" than when we hit puberty? **Aging changes bod-**

ies. Babies don't look like toddlers. Preteens don't look like twentysomethings. Sixty-year-olds *should* look different from thirty-year-olds.

Google has millions of articles on how women's bodies change. But I didn't have to swipe to the second page of results before I found articles that added helpful information on "what to do about it." The marketing narrative sells the story that living, eating, and exercising "right" keeps your body preserved like a jar of pickles. You'll never age, never gain weight. Fear and shame-inducing messages and "ten ways to turn back the hands of time" articles make you feel your body is a problem in need of a solution. But maybe, it's just a normal body. *Maybe a changing body isn't the enemy.*

Instead, we have a real enemy who seeks to steal, kill, and destroy. **What if one of his easiest attacks is to keep us distracted by our changing bodies, believing the lies and spending countless dollars and hours focused on a makeover mission instead of God's purpose for our lives?** *Hmm* . . .

Body Kindness

Yes, aging feels uncomfortable. Body changes are difficult to navigate. But what if, instead of trying to find ways to be rescued from the realities of a body that is (according to 2 Corinthians 4:16) wasting away, we could determine to befriend our body *through* these changes? What if instead of stressing over gaining weight, we could gain *wait*—the patience to endure the shifts of aging? What if we postured our hearts and minds to be gentle with these physical vessels we've been given? **Befriending and being kind to our bodies could be the most radical thing we do for our health.**

But What about Health?

When we talk about body struggles, this "h" word can tangle us up like old necklaces in a jewelry box. Many women say that they're afraid if they *don't* change how they look, they won't be healthy. Yet when asked, "If your appearance never changed yet the doctor gave you a clean bill of health, would you be satisfied?" they say no. It's hard to believe that health isn't a jeans size. Rather, health is a combination of factors—emotional, spiritual, mental, and physical. There's no body type, size, or look that has the monopoly on health.

Even if you're convinced you'll feel better after you lose some weight or fix some parts, understand that the truck goes before the trailer. Until you are secure in whose image you are made, it's difficult to feel secure in your body or free enough in your relationship with food to make healthy changes. **We need to come to the place where we're more afraid of not letting ourselves grow than we are of letting ourselves go.**

We Need a Hero

Yes, the fear is real. But it's helpful to remember, once again, who's behind the fearmongering. It's not God who dictates that we do whatever it takes to look youthful and spry. Those demands come from constructs of culture that want us to conform—often so that they can get wealthy. **But God didn't mess up when he allowed for aging.** He designed our bodies for this life. Note: He is the *only* one who can ask us to change with purely unselfish motives.

All concerns over our health, our appearance, our aging bodies are solved through remembering who rescues us. Drawing closer to God is the only way to feel the truth that we are safe to trust him with every concern. His Word says we can hide in the shelter of his wings (Psalm 91:4). He will never leave us or forsake us (Deuteronomy 31:8). He is our strong tower (Proverbs 18:10). The fear that lingers underneath our body image struggles can only be assuaged by a true Savior, a true hero, the only one with lasting solutions—that is Jesus.

Work It Out

Look up the three verses from the paragraph above or do your own Bible search for the words protection *and* secure. *What do you observe about how God keeps us safe and secure?*

What does it mean to you that the fear of the Lord is the fear to conquer all other fears?

Act

Prayer for Breaking Free from Fear

Dear Heavenly Father,

Forgive me for allowing fear to drive me to the worship of idols or to find security in people or things that are not you. Forgive me, Father, for the ways fear has propelled me to things I should not have pursued or paused me from pursuits that you ordained. I confess today that I haven't fully trusted you. Lord, as the father in Mark 9 called out, I believe, but help my unbelief! Today, I confess my perfectionism, my fear of the future, and my fear of what others will think or say about me. God, I confess the fears I've had related to my own opinions of myself and my fears of being misunderstood or wrongly judged by those around me. Help me to define my value by your Word alone and to tune out all other voices that push me to derive value from my body or appearance. Thank you for freeing me from all the ways I practice fear—from anxiety, control, and seeking approval.

In Jesus's name I pray. Amen.

Day 25

Get Thin, Fast

The spiritual discipline of fasting

The Pharisee stood by himself and prayed: "God, I thank you that I am not like other people.... I fast twice a week and give a tenth of all I get."

Luke 18:11–12

I was working in Washington, D.C., on Capitol Hill when I discovered the practice of Lent. Raised in the evangelical world, I'd never heard of this practice of denying oneself for forty days before Easter. This *had* to be the perfect diet. Imagine how awesome my willpower could be if I was giving up my favorite foods *for* God. I could get skinny *and* be a better Christian! *Win-win.*

In an office full of practicing Catholics, Lent would be easy. Several gave up sugar, which meant they'd stop bringing donuts on Fridays. Sugar-free was my best bet. My love of an afternoon frozen yogurt stood like an iceberg in the path of my smooth cruise to Thin Land. *This was such a good idea.*

So I gave up sugar. Completely. Even ketchup and barbeque sauce. *Good-bye, my loves.* I was the best "fast-er" around. After all, I was an experienced dieter. Restriction, deprivation—I had master's degrees in these subjects.

I fasted so well, I didn't stop when Easter came. This is what type-A overachievers do. I officially broke my "fast" on my birthday—in July!—with a slice of Cheesecake Factory's finest. I was so proud of my accomplishment. Oh, yes, and I did remember to pray some of those days too. *Yay!*

Biblical fasting is a beautiful spiritual discipline where we are to deny our bodies of food for the express purpose of drawing closer to God. The hunger we experience while fasting reminds us to hunger and thirst for righteousness. We fast to become full—full of God's love, grace, and humility. **Fasting allows us to lay down our desires and seek God without distraction.**

But that's not what I did anytime I engaged in fasting during my decades of dieting. I fear that diet culture has co-opted this spiritual discipline. Understand that any fast that promises "body results" is a diet. Any regiment where, after completion, you include the words, "Plus, I lost weight and look great!" may conflate the truth of Scripture with the propaganda of diet culture.

Follow me here. **If we're fasting to change how we look, how are we different from the Pharisee who fasted so others could see the brilliance of his spirituality?** If any part of our motivation is selfish or vain, can we really classify our deprivation as a spiritual discipline?

What has been your past relationship with fasting? Have you gone on fasts?

How have they felt like spiritually sacred times and/or how have they felt like diets?

How Did Daniel Fast?

A popular fasting model for Americans has been the fruits and vegetables fast—modeled after what Daniel and his friends did in Daniel chapter 1. Daniel and his friends were smart and handsome and were drafted for service in the house of the king. Note: Their people were in captivity. These Jewish boys didn't have a choice about where they'd work. Being obstinate in the king's palace could send you to the gallows or, at best, back to a less desirable form of labor.

The king ordered these men be trained for three years and groomed for service. He assigned them meals and beverages and put his chief official in charge of their regiment.

But Daniel had religious convictions about what they were asked to eat. His concern, in verse 8, is that the food would defile them. The Babylonians commonly ate pig and horse—both of which were forbidden for Jews. Other foods may have been offered to the gods of Babylon, and food offered to idols was also deemed unclean for Daniel.[1]

Some speculate that Daniel's real reason for refusing to eat the king's meatballs and Merlot may not be about the food at all. Sharing meals represented a depth of commitment and symbolized a kindred relationship. Did Daniel want to make it clear that his true loyalty remained with God and not the king of Babylon? What if, by not eating the king's offerings, Daniel symbolically demonstrated that he was dependent on God alone?[2]

Daniel says they won't eat the goods, and the chief pushes back on Daniel's conviction. He'll lose his job if these guys following Daniel look weak and skinny. But Daniel (with the Lord's favor) asks for a ten-day test run. He does the unthinkable, asking the chief to do a side-by-side comparison at the end of the trial. Daniel is so confident that God will honor their food decisions, he bets his body on it.

At the end of the test period, Daniel and his friends looked healthier and better nourished. So the chief official allowed them to continue eating this way—one would presume for the entire three years they were in preparation for the king's service.

They Got Fatter?

When you read that last paragraph through the lens of diet culture, it seems clear. We're getting dieting advice from God on high! *We should all become vegetarians! It's biblical!* But friend, don't stop reading here lest you miss important context.

Other translations of Daniel 1:15 (ESV) say that at the end of the ten days, it was seen that these men were "better in appearance and fatter in flesh than all the youths who ate the king's food." Cutting meat and dairy made them fatter? *What a tragic disappointment if you were hoping to see your results on the scale!*

But we need to understand that, culturally, thin wasn't in. In fact, if you were thin, it was because you were poor and couldn't afford to eat well. It was

1. Phillip J. Long, "Daniel 1:8–16—What Was Wrong with the King's Food?" Reading Acts, January 23, 2020, https://readingacts.com/2020/01/23/daniel-18-16-what-was-wrong-with-the-kings-food/.
    2. Long, "Daniel 1:8–16—What Was Wrong with the King's Food?"

important that the king's men not look like the undernourished masses. Being plump was a way to show your wealth and privilege.

It should also be noted that their diet likely included bread. Susan Weingarten explains that bread was such a common staple of everyone's diet that it didn't need a special callout in the text. And while many English translations of the Bible interpret the Hebrew word for *seed* as *vegetables*, Jerome, when completing the Vulgate, translated it as *legumina*—legumes or pulses. These are in the bean and pea family—each would provide protein these teenage boys needed.[3]

After three years of lentil soup, for Daniel's posse to look fatter or fuller in any way is nothing short of a miracle. God put his hand of favor and protection on these boys pledging their allegiance to God alone. **Their decision to refrain from certain foods was not about the foods, the temptation of the foods, or the way they would look afterward.** There wasn't an ounce of vanity involved in their decision to fast. Instead, they may have begged God to not let the impact of fasting show up on their physical bodies.

This truly is the only way to keep the purpose of our fasts spiritual. Otherwise, our temptation is to, like the Pharisees, "show off" the results of our fast.

Work It Out

Read Matthew 6:16. How do you think Jesus's words about fasting for other people to see may relate to fasting for transformation?

Imagine how it would feel to deny yourself food for forty days and see no physical change in your body. What thoughts come to mind when you consider fasting for the spiritual benefit only?

---

3. Susan Weingarten, "Food in Daniel 1:5–16: The First Report of a Controlled Experiment?" The James Lind Library, 2018, https://www.jameslindlibrary.org/articles/food-daniel-15-16-first-report-controlled-experiment/.

Read Mark 10:28-31. As you think about fasting, what differences do you see between temporarily giving up food for the cause of Christ and giving up food for a thinner body?

Spiritual Discipline Versus Eating Disorders

As someone with a disordered eating background, I may never be able to fast the way God intended. I'm still attempting to add boundaries so I can fast without making it a diet. Now I ask friends to keep me accountable. The minute my thoughts turn to how flat my stomach feels or how thin I could be after a few more weeks of restricting food, that's my cue that I'm no longer fasting for Jesus.

Day 26

Living in the Grace

Letting go of black-and-white thinking

> Whatever keeps me from the Bible is my enemy, however harmless it may appear to be.
>
> *A.W. Tozer*

There's one question I get asked every time I speak: Where's the line between stewarding my body well and body image idolatry?

The answer is found in the Matthew 6 treasure principle. In the Sermon on the Mount, Jesus teaches that where your treasure is, your heart will be also. The principle here isn't just about money or earthly possessions. Beauty, body image, food rules, exercise regiments—these things can easily become treasures we seek instead of Jesus. In verses 19 and 20 we read, "Do not store up for yourselves treasures on earth, where moths and vermin destroy, and where thieves break in and steal. But store for yourselves treasures in heaven. . . ."

Think of money. There's not a point when an alarm sounds to signal you've transformed from a good steward to Ebenezer Scrooge. **Similarly, no bell dings when you cross over from caring for your body to making your body's appearance or health the central focus of your life.** It requires being honest with yourself and being willing to daily submit this subject to God and listen for the Holy Spirit's input.

If your bank account is suffering from what you've spent on body improvement, it may be time to consider the possibility that this could be an idol in your life. Likewise, if you spend copious amounts of time at the gym, meal prepping, thinking about diets and macros, or otherwise fixated on body change, it's likely that you've put body change, body image, or body improvement in too lofty a position. If what you can't live without is your daily run, not your daily quiet time, take this opportunity for self-evaluation.

Living in the Gray

"Don't make beauty your treasure . . ." is a difficult answer for those of us who prefer things to be black and white. We're more comfortable living with rules, checking boxes, and following a plan. We want to know what it takes to be righteous. We're the ones who enjoyed getting report cards in school. It's nice to know *exactly* how you're doing.

Remember, the Pharisees felt the same way. They were unnerved by Jesus and his teachings about what happens in one's heart as being equal to what one actually does. Hating someone because she's skinnier than me is the same as murder? *Surely not.*

But the Christian life isn't like other religions. We have freedom to be led by our Holy Spirit–filled consciences and to make choices based on what is most loving to those around us. I'd call it living in the gray, but that's not really accurate. That could be misconstrued as some sort of dismissal of principles of right and wrong. So instead, I'll call it living in the grace.

What is Black-and-White Thinking?

Black-and-white thinking is also called all-or-nothing thinking or splitting. Essentially, it's a struggle to see things realistically—a cognitive distortion where we fail to mentally bring together positive and negative aspects of ourselves, others, or our circumstances. Life feels terrible or wonderful. Friends are classified besties one day and mortal enemies the next. We're either perfect or complete failures. There's no in-between.

Absolutes and extremes characterize black-and-white thinking. Here are some of the words one may use that fall into the category of black-and-white thinking.

Circle the words you find yourself using in daily life:

Always	Failure	Should
Never	Success	Ought
Impossible	All	Disaster
Ruined	Nothing	It's Over
Perfect	Amazing	Awful

In the context of body image, black-and-white thinking motivates us to classify foods as good or bad, look at our bodies as disgusting or almost perfect, and/or eat in binge-purge cycles where extreme restriction will be followed by binges that are then followed by restriction again. From a biblical perspective, we are saints who wrestle sin (Romans 6:12). **We're new creations who battle our old ways. The dissonance between who we are and who we want to be is what leads us to God's grace.** His kindness leads us to repentance. Seeing myself as all bad even after salvation isn't accurate. Likewise, seeing myself as better than I am isn't in line with Paul's admonition in Romans 12:3 to consider myself with sober judgment.

Breaking Black-and-White Thinking Patterns

Psychologists recommend a variety of tactics for dealing with black-and-white thinking, from mindfulness and meditation to intentionally telling yourself a different story when you spiral into all-or-nothing despair. But the gospel gives us hope to completely rewrite the narratives in our head under the umbrella of God's grace.

Identify your feelings in each thought, but recognize that feelings aren't always based on truth. In other words: Don't believe everything you think. Sometimes we can "feel" like a friend is ignoring us because she hasn't responded to a text message when, truthfully, she's been sick or handling a family crisis. Every feeling we have must go through the filter of Philippians 4:8 (ESV): "Whatever is true, whatever is honorable, whatever is just, whatever is pure, whatever is lovely, whatever is commendable, if there is any excellence, if there is anything worthy of praise, think about these things." There are facts and there are feelings. They often aren't the same. Being able to tell the difference between the two is essential to overcoming black-and-white thinking.

Black-and-White Thinking Versus Grace-Filled Thinking

"I never eat like I'm supposed to eat."	"According to whom? I'm free to enjoy a variety of foods."
"I should exercise more."	"I feel like I should exercise more, but I'm free to joyfully move my body whenever I'm able."
"My body is ruined."	"My body is always changing to help me stay alive. I'm made in God's image. I won't condemn my body; I'll care for it."
"I always fail when I try to get healthier. I'll never get it right."	"Staying on a plan is not the same as getting healthier. I am free to add healthy, sustainable habits without the guilt and shame of trying to follow a man-made plan perfectly."

Living in the Grace with Your Body

An all-or-nothing approach is detrimental to every area of your health. This is a common pitfall for dieters. We're either all in or all out. On the plan or off the wagon. Black-and-white thinking keeps us from moving our bodies unless we have time for a full workout session. When we know the diet starts Monday, it's harder to honor our fullness on Sunday night.

Obsessing over being a perfect wife, mom, daughter, or employee never consumed the same amount of mental space for me as obsessing over being a "perfect" eater or having "perfect" workout weeks. But even conceptualizing that someone could be perfect in the arena of caring for their body is black-and-white thinking. "Perfect" eaters and "perfect" bodies don't exist (this side of heaven, at least). **Just like none of us are perfect stewards of our time or our money, we all struggle to steward our bodies "perfectly."** But black-and-white thinking drives us to miss the opportunity to just be good stewards (as Scripture instructs) and trust the rest to God's grace.

Work It Out

Read Philippians 4:8. How would running your thoughts about your body through this filter change the way you speak or think about your body?

In what areas do you default to black-and-white thinking? List your most frequent "always" and "never" thoughts here.

Read 2 Corinthians 12:9; 2 Corinthians 9:8; and 1 Corinthians 15:10. What principles of grace can you apply to your body image struggle?

Act

Memorize Philippians 4:8.

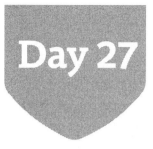

Day 27

Covering Shame

Finding emotional health

> Unless you stole it, you should never feel guilty about any food you eat.
>
> *Anonymous*

I just spent fifteen minutes thinking of all the ways I'm better than someone else. It's tragic, really. *Help me, Lord.* But it happened so naturally I didn't recognize the path my brain had taken until I arrived there. I judged another woman to be excelling in one area of life more than I am, so to make myself feel better, my thoughts instantly hopped to all the ways I had one up on her until I could congratulate myself for winning the imaginary contest. *Ugh.*

As embarrassing as it is for me to share that with you, I want to, because I have a feeling you do it too. You see her Instagram picture. You think of the ways she's getting ahead of you. Then you self-soothe by recounting all the other ways in which you are better. It's ugly. And it's all hidden. These are the secret judgments we cast and then keep to ourselves.

Our brains do this to protect us. It is discouraging to sit around thinking everyone's getting ahead, so our brains may just be trying to keep us from falling into the downward spiral of depression. How we coach ourselves in these situations often depends on how our parents talked to us when we felt we weren't measuring up. If our parents always deflected our feelings of defeat and focused on the ways we were competing well, it only makes sense that this path has been burned into our neural pathways.

Shame and Pride

It's strange, but I look at pictures from my fittest days and I know I felt far more shame twenty years ago wearing a much smaller size than I do now. I can hardly believe the woman in those old photos obsessed so much over her body. Anything you put under a magnifying glass gets bigger.

Though shame and pride seem like opposites, both keep us focused on ourselves above all else. Both wield tremendous power over our emotional lives. It may seem like the proud person wouldn't struggle with shame, but this couldn't be further from the truth. Shame can't exist without pride. And too often, those who get stuck wallowing in shame are really stuck wallowing in pride—wanting to believe they are good enough on their own.

If you've ever battled perfectionist tendencies, you may understand. The feeling that you're never enough, that you are constantly missing your high mark, or that you are failing to meet your own standards or the standards of others can be debilitating. **The more "perfect" one becomes in their projected image to the world, the more the pressure builds to maintain this image.** And the more failure, disappointment, and shame the one wearing this burden feels when they can't keep up the act.

An emotionally healthy person accepts both their strengths and weaknesses. They face mistakes, failures, and miscalculations as a normal part of life and being human. But for the perfectionist, the shame of not meeting their own high standard weighs heavy. Weaknesses go on the "to be fixed" checklist.

It's mental trickery. We believe that if our bodies were better, we would be proud of them—not ashamed. We'd be posting bikini pictures on social media (or, at least we'd know we could if we wanted to). **But body pride has no power to cure body shame. Only Jesus can do that.**

The Holy Grail of Body Image Freedom

Like Indiana Jones, my quest was to find the Holy Grail of body transformation. There's no site I wouldn't excavate, no stone I wouldn't overturn to find the plan to free me from this struggle. What I really longed for wasn't freedom from the "wrong" number on the scale but from my shame.

Shame shakes its finger, saying we've "messed up," then never stops condemning. Though guilt is often confused with shame, guilt connects to actions, while shame relates to identity. We carry shame in deep, hidden places, believing that we're flawed because of these feelings.

Author Karen Koenig explains that how we've learned to handle our shame comes from our families of origin. If you were taught that all people make mistakes—and were allowed to make them and move on—there's a good chance shame doesn't plague you much. But if you were constantly reminded of or labeled by your mistakes, or conversely, if you were never allowed to feel your mistakes by parents who tried to protect you from disappointment or rejection—both can cause us to have a heightened sense of shame.[1] Perhaps you were subtly shamed by parents who thought they were encouraging you to look and be your best. But instead, their efforts were interpreted as criticism that laid the groundwork for future perfectionism. Maybe you learned that there was always something else to improve before you could be deemed acceptable.

Or maybe you were directly shamed for your size or food choices. To be caught with forbidden foods was akin to getting caught stealing. Were you told that your body was unacceptable? Maybe you were forced to diet, step on a scale, or stare at "undesirable" body parts in the mirror with Mom, Dad, or Grandma's scrutiny. All of these experiences can cause deep shame. It hurts to experience these subtle or overt rejections of your body.

But you'll never be perfect enough to cure the shame. Neither can you ever go back and prove worthiness to the one who shamed you. It doesn't work that way. The power of their cruel words will always hold a grip on your heart until you surrender the shame to the only one who can completely cover it—Jesus.

Maybe your parents tried to protect you from ever experiencing shame. They coddled and made you feel like you were already perfect, even if others didn't recognize it. Koenig explains how parents who always deflect shame make us feel like we aren't equipped to handle it. Instead of saving us from feeling shame, we instead feel double.[2] The super-perfectionist is born!

---

1. Karen R. Koenig, *The Food and Feelings Workbook: A Full Course Meal on Emotional Health* (Carlsbad: Gürze Books, 2007), 86–89.
2. Koenig, *The Food and Feelings Workbook*, 89.

We determine to fight shame by winning. Once we reach the top, no one can touch us. We'll be safe from the shame then, we believe. No one criticizes the winner, right?

Yet there's no anecdotal evidence for this anywhere. The better we do, the more critical we become. The more we perfect our bodies, the more we zoom in on every minor flaw. Koenig writes, "Perfectionism feeds on itself—the more you fear the shame of imperfection, the more perfect you have to be."[3] We can never be free from body shame until we recognize its connection to pride.

What are some ways you feel or experience shame around your body or body-change choices now?

On a scale of 1–10, how desperate do you feel to be free from shame that is related to your body or body-change choices?

1 · · · · · 2 · · · · · 3 · · · · · 4 · · · · · 5 · · · · · 6 · · · · · 7 · · · · · 8 · · · · · 9 · · · · · 1 0

I don't feel shame.   I sometimes feel shame.   Shame overwhelms me.

Work It Out

Pause and think about how you encountered shame as a child. Were you criticized? Made to feel like you weren't good enough? Teased or picked on? Were there specific areas of achievement or appearance that family members criticized you about?

3. Koenig, *The Food and Feelings Workbook*, 93.

Were you allowed to feel the consequences of mistakes you made, or were you taught to do better next time? Or were you told you weren't the problem—those who were making you feel the shame needed to do better?

Both pride and shame invoke many irrational beliefs. Circle some irrational beliefs you've held:

I should be ashamed of the way I eat.

I should be ashamed of my weight.

I don't deserve what other people deserve because of my appearance.

I should be ashamed when I don't get to exercise.

I should be ashamed of my skin.

I should be ashamed of my height or build.

I should be ashamed if clothes from years ago don't fit.

I should feel ashamed that my body has changed.

I should be ashamed of the signs of aging.

I should be ashamed that I look my age.

I don't deserve what other people have because of the way my body looks.

What would you add to this list?

Act

Shame thrives in the secret but struggles to survive when it's shared. Shining the light on shame happens best in community, where we can be reminded that nothing we struggle with is unique to us and, similarly, nothing we wrestle is surprising to Jesus. Here are some ways to begin releasing shame.

Mark one and commit to trying it soon.

- ☐ Write a letter to your spouse or a trusted friend sharing how you struggle with shame.

- ☐ Sit down with someone you trust and share one way that you feel bogged down by shame.

- ☐ Write a letter to Jesus, spelling out all the ways you feel ashamed and asking him to take this shame from you.

- ☐ Invite a few women to read through and discuss this book with you. When you get to this chapter, share openly the ways you struggle with shame and watch how you free other women to do the same.

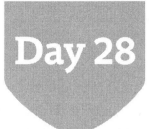

Day 28

How Then Shall We Eat?

Spiritually healthy ways to relate to food and body

Listen to your body. It's smarter than you.

Anonymous

Years ago, I spoke at a women's event here in Austin where the breakfast buffet table made it evident this was a "crunchy" group. I grabbed what looked to be an organic brownie bar and some fruit and made my way to a table. The brownie appeared chocolaty, but I could tell a whole lot of trendy health ingredients had been jammed in there too. I broke it open to get a better look, when something crawled out of the brownie and across my plate! No matter how nutrient dense that little creature was, I suddenly lost my appetite.

One of the things I love most about when women gather is that there's usually delicious food involved. But what I hate is how diet culture has made everyone feel like they should apologize for enjoying it (or bringing it!). *I'm so sorry, I was going to make the fat-free, gluten-free, sugar-free version, but I ran out of time.*

Where did our relationship with food go astray? As we explored several days ago, diet culture's influence has convoluted the Bible's teaching on feasting, fasting, and everything in between. If we can't trust the latest diet craze, how do we know what to eat? How to exercise? How to define health? *I can tell you for sure, if this "added bugs" trend catches on, I'm out.*

Here are some snapshot answers to these questions you can reference whenever you're feeling confused about how to relate in these areas.

How Do We Eat?

We ask God for the grace to help us make wise decisions for our bodies, one day at a time, one meal at a time. We allow ourselves the freedom Christ has granted us to enjoy foods that satisfy and nourish us, without adding guilt and shame over rules that were created by man and are subject to change. We eat regularly so that our bodies can work as God intended them to. Similarly, we understand our responsibility to tend to our body's needs with nutrients but refuse to become enslaved to food rules. When eating in the presence of others, we seek peace and embrace hospitality to avoid the pitfalls of the gluttony of delicacy. We make decisions about food based on what is most loving to those we are with (Romans 14).

(If relating to food in this way is too uncomfortable, seek professional help to restore and heal your relationship with food.)

Write one sentence about how you would like to relate to food:

How Do We Exercise?

Exercise looks like joyful movement. Its purpose is not to pay penance for perceived food sins or to burn off more calories than we've eaten to reach a desired body size or shape. Neither do we exercise to bring more glory to our bodies or to draw praise for ourselves that belongs to God alone. Instead, the mental and physical health benefits of exercise can be freely enjoyed and acknowledged as outlets that keep us fit to serve the King, not ourselves. We seek to move our bodies in ways that honor God and make us feel healthy and strong (1 Timothy 4:8). We best enjoy the blessing of mobility by using our bodies as instruments of worship.

Write one sentence about how you would like to relate to exercise:

How Do We Think about Our Bodies?

We acknowledge that our bodies are good. They were made by God for his good purposes. We don't have to get high on body love or trash our bodies like a hotel room we'll check out of after our years on earth. Instead, we respect how God created our bodies by listening to cues like hunger and fullness, injury, or exhaustion. We remember what Romans 12 says—our bodies are a living sacrifice. We will choose to make them holy, acceptable, and pleasing to God, even if that means something different from shaping or sculpting them to please others or ourselves! I take care of my body because it is a gift from a God who loves me.

Write one sentence about how you would like to think about your body:

How Do We Think about Our Health?

Living in grace means we make the best decisions we can for our health without becoming preoccupied or consumed with the quest for optimal health. We do what we can, and we trust God to care for us even more than we trust our supplements, treatments, doctors, and wellness plans. We recognize that health can become an idol just as easily as money or beauty, and we acknowledge that no matter how much health we achieve, our bodies are only temporary (2 Corinthians 4:16). To have a healthy body at the expense of cultivating a healthy, surrendered, and pure heart before God would be a loss, not gain.

Write one sentence about how you would like to relate to your health:

Work It Out

Take a few minutes to reread the sentences you wrote above about how you'd like to relate to food and exercise and how you'd like to think about your body and your health. What is one thing you can do today to put into practice each of these goals?

One thing I can do to improve how I relate to food is:

One thing I can do to improve how I relate to exercise is:

One thing I can do to improve how I think about my body is:

One thing I can do to improve how I think about health is:

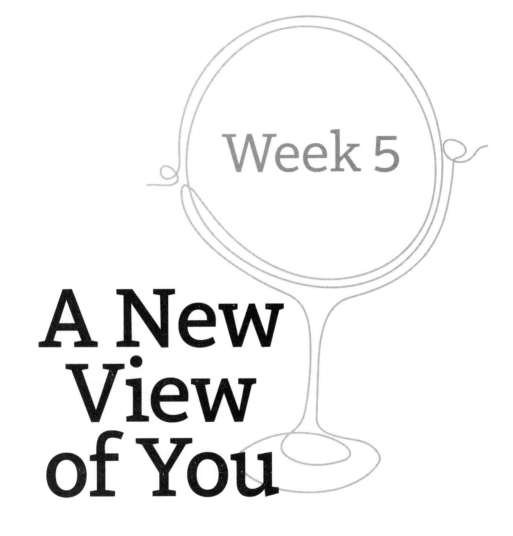

Week 5

A New View of You

A Closet Full of Grief

Letting go of your ideal body

> The darker the night, the brighter the stars,
> The deeper the grief, the closer is God!
>
> *Fyodor Dostoevsky*

My friend Dana from *A Slob Comes Clean* joined me on my podcast a few years ago. She's a home organizing expert, and we talked about why so many women (like me) who struggle with body image issues have a hard time cleaning old clothes out of our closets. Her answer shocked me. She called it grief!

Grief? I do prefer wearing black, but no one's died. I thought it was slimming.

Dana's words stuck. As I spoke with women about their ideal bodies and how many years (or decades) they'd been striving to attain that ideal, I realized that the problem Dana spotted wasn't just in our closets. It's in our hearts. And it needs to come out.

Now I take my clients through an important exercise to grieve the loss of that ideal. For some, the grief connects to aging and changing, accepting they'll never have the body of a thirty-year-old again. In other cases, especially with younger clients, we grieve the loss of an ideal body they've never achieved so they can sit in the grace of reality. Living for these ideals distracts them from living for Jesus. Likewise, the pursuit of these ideals (remember—a synonym for *idols*) may keep us from God's best.

Grieving the Ideal Me

In a culture where there's an eight-week course to fix your every problem, it's hard to believe a struggle-free existence isn't just a few tweaks away.

Yet even if I can wear a smaller size or get my hair to cooperate, there's no permanence to our current physical beings. I may feel content for a few weeks or months, but as things start shifting again, any confidence placed in my "new and improved" body will wane. In fact, research shows that women who have gone through these kinds of body changes find themselves even more body-focused after the change than they were before. Instead of the body change freeing them, those chains got heavier.[1]

Limiting Beliefs

Limiting beliefs are patterns in our thinking that are so well-worn, it's hard for us to accept that anything else could be true. *Of course I'll feel better once I lose the weight! Of course I'll be excited to wear a swimsuit once I've sculpted my abs! How could I not like the way I look in pictures after I get my body just the way I want it to look?*

Ahh . . . but even models don't like the way they look in pictures. And while waiting to achieve a better body, how many of those photo opportunities do we step out of? I wrestled every year scheduling a family photo session. I didn't feel "ready" to be in the pictures. But as I waited, hoping to change my body, time didn't stop. In fact, there are a few precious years of my children's lives where we don't have nice family photos because I wasn't ready to be in them! Those children, they just kept growing. And I'll never have a chance to go back and capture that moment in time with them at that age and stage.

That's what limiting beliefs do. **As we wait for "someday," we miss out on now, trapped in an if/then paradigm.** Instead of planning that vacation, applying for that job, volunteering at church, or getting back to the dating scene, we put our lives on hold until we get our bodies "fixed." Yet I work with clients in their sixties and seventies who fight gravity as they continue their quest for an improved body. **If you're waiting for life to start after you get your ideal body, you may never get a chance to live it.**

---

1. Alice G. Walton, "Slimming Down Might Not Improve Your Body Image," *The Atlantic*, May 3, 2012, https://www.theatlantic.com/health/archive/2012/05/slimming-down-might-not-improve-your-body-image/256726/.

Stages of Grieving

Can we delicately and without despair surrender these dreams with open hands to God? Though it may feel like a death in the family, God will be faithful to help us process the loss and find a new way to live. It takes courage. It takes faith. But in addition to freedom, you may gain closet space. *I'm guessing I'm not the only one who holds on to clothes that no longer fit.*

Elisabeth Kübler-Ross created a framework for understanding how we process loss, which she called the Five Stages of Grief: denial, anger, bargaining, depression, and acceptance.[2] Let's briefly look at each of these stages in the context of our body image.

Denial: This is the most difficult hurdle to clear for most women who have been in pursuit of a better body. It's hard to accept that I don't have complete control over my body's shape or size (especially when diet culture tells us otherwise). Releasing the dream that "someday I will look like I want to look and everything will be better" hurts.

Anger: Many of my clients feel angry that they've wasted time and money trying to change their bodies yet still feel dissatisfied. Sometimes accompanying this anger is frustration at industries and marketers who have kept them spending and yo-yo-ing. Or they're angry at others who seem caught up in the body change game. Scripture reminds us, "Be angry and do not sin . . ." (Ephesians 4:26 ESV). Though blaming or condemning others will never free us, reaching an "enough is enough" attitude can help us shift our thinking away from believing that a better body can save us.

Bargaining: This is the stage where we "woulda, shoulda, coulda" our way through the past as we examine "what would my body have been like if I had . . . or if I hadn't . . ." Sitting in bargaining can feel uncomfortable, theologically, as we bring questions to God about our past, his sovereignty over that past, and the choices we made for ourselves.

Depression: Many women who wrestle body image issues struggle with depression and anxiety. They are often unaware that the depression they battle accompanies loss. Depressed feelings connect to ideals and dreams that were never fulfilled. When the fortieth diet doesn't work, or the latest magic

---

2. Elisabeth Kübler-Ross, *On Death and Dying* (New York: Simon & Schuster/Collier Books, 1970).

supplement doesn't clear your skin, sadness is a reasonable response. **I encourage clients to be honest with God about their disappointment and to lament.** Depressed feelings can set the stage for us to finally be ready to come to God, confess the image idol, repent, and then feel his grace and love gently nudge us toward a new path. (Please talk to a professional if your depression is affecting your daily ability to function.)

Acceptance: Acceptance—in any type of grief—doesn't mean that you never miss the person (or the dream). Instead, it means you've bravely faced your new reality and can move forward, despite the loss you feel. For the Christian overcoming body image issues, acceptance can look like learning to live more fully in your body, practicing body kindness, and expressing gratitude, even if you're not convinced you like your body yet.

Grief Doesn't Follow a Set Pattern

Understand, grief isn't linear. You may not experience the stages in this order, or you may bounce back and forth between two stages before moving to another. If you've ever lost someone close to you, you know how grief can surprise you. You can go from feeling fine to being flooded with memories in a matter of seconds. Grieving your ideal body may feel the same way. You may be walking through a store you once shopped in and feel a sudden flood of sadness over not being the age or size you used to be. Without notice, you may find yourself working through bargaining, depression, anger, denial, and acceptance again.

Grieving your ideal body is worth the pain. This is the path to body acceptance —understanding that God gave you your body on purpose and for His purpose. I can't wait for you to see how amazing it is to feel good in your own skin.

Work It Out

What stages of grief do you believe you've experienced in your body image journey?

Look at these psalms of lament: Psalm 12, Psalm 22, Psalm 13, and Psalm 44. What do you notice about the way the psalmist pours his heart out to God? Can you relate to his laments?

Write your own lament over your ideal body here:

Act

You have two options for actions you can take today as you process body grief.

Option 1: Schedule a photo session. If you've been putting off getting family photos or professional headshots, schedule this today. Pray that God will help you grieve the loss of how you would "ideally" look in these photos and give you the grace and peace to accept the real you, just as you are, when the pictures are taken.

Option 2: Pull out a few items of clothing hanging in your closet or lingering in your drawers that don't fit. Hold each garment and thank God for any good memories you have of wearing it. Thank him for that season of your life and ask him to give you the grace to accept this new season you are in. Then donate or sell these garments.

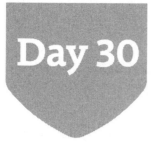

Day 30

Pinching an Inch

Body checking and living embodied

> Some people, no matter how old they get, never lose their beauty—they merely move it from their faces to their hearts.
>
> *Martin Buxbaum*

"Thanks to the K, you can't pinch an inch on me!"

In 1984, Kellogg's decided to promote Special K cereal as diet food. Some ads featured a man squeezing a bit of flesh from above his wife's tiny waist. Don't worry. She pinched him back around the middle until they both determined to eat more Special K! *Insert eye roll here.* A few years later, the concept turned into a jingle. "If you can pinch an inch," the ad proclaimed, "you should eat more Special K!" Beyond how hokey this sounds, can you imagine cereal being marketed as a diet food now?

If, like me, you were raised watching these commercials, you may have learned to test your body size through this pinching practice. Many of my clients have been subconsciously doing it for decades. Even if you were never exposed to ridiculous 1980s cereal ads, you may have your own methods of feeling or checking your body.

Body Checking

Body checking is a compulsive habit for many who struggle with body image issues. Not all body checking is unhealthy, of course. Making sure there's no toothpaste on your face and that your clothing is all zipped and buttoned up is not harmful. But for some, body checking doesn't confine itself to morning getting-ready rituals. Every time there's reflective glass, the compulsive body checker must check to see how they're doing. Anxiety surges for these men and women as they fixate on what they see or feel and get caught up in an unhealthy headspace for minutes or hours afterward based on the feedback.

Data suggests that body checking often leaves you feeling worse about your body.[1] In fact, the more you stare at your stomach or chin, the more you'll think about it and the more miserable you'll become. **No woman with body image issues ever walks away from a mirror encouraged.** The older you get, the more that magazine article advice to stare into the mirror until you find something you love sounds ludicrous.

A 2004 study showed that body checking is closely connected to disordered eating.[2] One looks to the mirror to give permission to eat more or eat what we crave, but the mirror gives an opposing message. Likewise, those with disordered eating can use the mirror to "check the damage" done after eating to see if the perceived harm done by consuming calories or a forbidden food has shown up on their body in an obvious way. Of course, this isn't how the body works, so any perception of body change after eating would just be in one's mind. But it's difficult to get the compulsive body checker to believe that.[3]

Body checking can be a part of a morning ritual, or you may subconsciously find yourself feeling around your stomach, face, arms, or legs to do the pinch test whenever you're feeling anxious, stressed, or worried. It's like our bodies are hoping to comfort themselves through reassurance that our bodies look or feel the way we want them to. But the checking often backfires and adds more stress.

---

1. Liliana Almeida, "What Is Body Checking?" Verywell Mind, updated March 22, 2022, https://www.verywell mind.com/reduce-body-checking-with-two-easy-steps-1138366.

2. Roz Shafran, Christopher G. Fairburn, Paul Robinson, and Bryan Lask, "Body Checking and Its Avoidance in Eating Disorders," *International Journal of Eating Disorders* 35, no. 1 (2004): 93–101, https://pubmed.ncbi.nlm.nih.gov/14705162/.

3. Rebecca Joy Stanborough, "What's Body Checking and How Can You Control It?" Healthline, October 16, 2020, https://www.healthline.com/health/body-checking.

The Illusion of Control

Body checking is about control. If you weigh yourself daily to "make sure it doesn't get out of hand," you may understand how control and body image issues closely connect.

Controlling the health of our bodies through trying to control their size is mere illusion. I know women who meet the cultural standard of the ideal size and have had knee and hip replacements, were diagnosed with rheumatoid arthritis or other autoimmune diseases, or faced cancer. Likewise, I know women with larger bodies with clean bills of health who've never so much as taken a prescription medicine.

Body checking to keep body size "managed" fuels eating disorders and disordered eating. Similarly, it disconnects us from developing a healthy relationship with our body as we worry about our appearance instead of living our lives to God's glory.

Here's What to Do If You're a Body Checker

1) Acknowledge that you have a body checking habit. Whether it's compulsive weighing or pinching your belly, notice the behavior, and begin to keep tabs on how often you do it. Seeing the problem is the first step to solving it.

2) Type out your favorite Scripture verse about your worth and value in Christ. Print it and put this piece of paper over the part of your mirror that you are most likely to check (for example, place it low if you check your stomach).

3) Consider a thirty-day mirror fast. In this fast, you're allowed to take a brief glance to make sure your makeup and clothes are on right, but don't linger there. Former model Jennifer Strickland did this fast while meditating on Psalm 34:5 (ESV): "Those who look to him are radiant, and their faces shall never be ashamed."

4) Break the habit of feeling your stomach, chin, thighs, or other body parts by creating a new habit of feeling something soft in your pocket or a necklace worn around your neck. Consider a cross necklace to remind you that you're still worthy. When you want to rub your hand over your stomach, rub the cross instead.

As we age and change, it becomes even more important to befriend our bodies—not fight them. In fact, studies show that the healthiest way to live is with a great attitude. How you feel about your life and your level of optimism and hope for the future matter more to your overall health than what you eat.[4] Other studies take this one step further. Those who have more hope for the future naturally engage in more body-healthy habits.[5]

Life in Person

Though it may seem like checking our bodies exemplifies awareness of being in them, it doesn't really work that way. Body checking is a form of objectification, while embodiment—becoming more aware of how we live, move, and inhabit our bodies—brings healing. **Embodiment simply means recognizing that God created us to experience life in these bodies—not outside of them.** As the world turns more virtual and relationships more commonly include online exchanges or sharing videos back and forth, we must stay in tune with our embodiment. Loneliness is an epidemic. Physical touch is critically important for our health and development. And those of us with body image issues may be most tempted of all to try to do life without anyone interacting with (or seeing) our bodies!

In isolation, the enemy has the opportunity to continue feeding us lies. *If they see you, they'll reject you,* he taunts. It's easy to convince ourselves after days, weeks, or months without real interactions that maybe we're better off alone. Similarly, the disassociation between our "image" and the "real us" can grow. Let's be honest: We can be anyone we want to be online, right?

You were created to be an image bearer, to reflect God's light with others you meet and serve—not just others you scroll past. Much frustration accompanies trying to live a virtual life. We miss out on connection when only a few of our senses are engaged. Smell, for example, has a powerful impact on our memories. Perhaps that's why zoom calls are rarely memorable. *It's hard to smell through a screen.*

4. Harvard Chan School Communications, "Optimism Lengthens Life, Study Finds," *The Harvard Gazette*, June 8, 2022, https://news.harvard.edu/gazette/story/2022/06/optimism-lengthens-life-study-finds/.

5. Fuschia Sirois, "Why Optimists Live Longer Than the Rest of Us," *The Washington Post*, July 3, 2022, https://www.washingtonpost.com/health/2022/07/03/optimistists-live-longer-why/.

Work It Out

How much of my life am I living virtually versus embodied?

Do I spend a lot of time on social media, video games (including those phone games!), television, or other screen-related pastimes?

What activities from the list below could I add to my life to help me feel my embodiment?

Act

Ideas for a More Embodied Life

- **Invite a friend to lunch.** Connecting with someone in person can be more life-giving than you may expect. It may feel awkward at first, but having real, in-the-flesh friends is helpful to our bodies, our minds, and our souls. Many women who struggle with body image issues feel alone or believe they are the only ones who struggle. Connecting with other women you enjoy spending time with is key.
- **Go to church.** Yes, I know you can watch it online in your pajamas, but just go if you're physically able. There's no comparison between church through the screen and worshiping in real life with other believers.
- **Do a media purge.** Unfollow people who post their fitness photos, and unfollow anyone who posts messages about value and worth (even subtle ones) that are contrary to what you know to be true. Assess below

what shows you are watching and how they make you feel. Yes, you may feel better when you think you look good—but you and I know that there's also a way to look good on the outside and feel awful on the inside. Let's stop believing that others' lives are perfect because they take great pictures.

- My favorite shows:

- How I feel about my body after I look at or watch . . .

- **Consider a media fast.** Consider making this a media-free week. Stay off social media, TV, and similar places where you'll get confusing messages about bodies and beauty. Load the Bible app or move it to a place on your phone near where your Facebook and Instagram apps are, and relocate those apps to a back page (or remove them from your phone for a week!). Retrain your thumb to fill those few minutes here and there with reading Scripture instead of scrolling. Try it for a week and see how less burdened you feel.

Note for Trauma Victims

Being fully in your body is harder for some. If you've experienced trauma of any kind, you may need extra support in this arena. Our bodies are smart. If they don't feel safe, they will respond in a way that seems to offer you protection. Therapies like EMDR (Eye Movement Desensitization and Reprocessing), Christian counseling, or trauma-informed counseling may be able to help you further explore why you struggle in your body and how you can gain new freedom to live embodied.

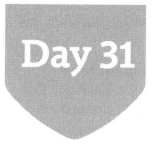

Day 31

The Greatest Love of All

How self-love distracts us

> But to be fully known and truly loved is, well, a lot like being loved by God. It is what we need more than anything. It liberates us from pretense, humbles us out of our self-righteousness, and fortifies us for any difficulty life can throw at us.
>
> *Tim Keller*

I was twelve years old—awkwardly approaching adolescence while clinging to the crumbs of childhood. My grandparents lived in downtown Harrisburg, Pennsylvania, and when we visited them, we'd play outside. Though I wasn't allowed to listen to secular music, that year I learned the song that dominated pop radio: "The Greatest Love of All" by Whitney Houston. Since sound effortlessly traveled from the adjacent houses into my grandparents' urban backyard, I heard the song repeatedly (must have been their neighbor's favorite) until I memorized some of the words. When the preteen me belted out the lyrics, I felt powerful!

Somewhere in my Sunday school–girl brain, I felt certain this song was about Jesus. Jesus was *obviously* the greatest love of all. This church song must've snuck onto mainstream radio. *Yay, team God!*

Until recently, while preparing for a talk on self-love, I discovered what Whitney really sang. She found the greatest love of all *inside* of her. But it wasn't Jesus. It was loving herself. *Interesting.*

Whitney crooned how she never found a hero to meet her needs. She learned to depend only on herself. The lyrics to this song feel especially tragic now, more than a decade after she drowned in a bathtub with her drug paraphernalia nearby. Her marriage misery had been tabloid fodder for decades. I'm deeply saddened for her. Did Whitney ever recognize that *her* greatest love of all wasn't enough?

What have you believed or been taught about self-love?

Have you ever felt like finding self-love would help you feel better about your body?

Self-Love and the Gospel

In the 1940s, psychologist Abraham Maslow created a hierarchy of human needs to theorize a path as to how people can live to their truest potential.

The pinnacle of human existence, according to Maslow, is self-actualization. Though Maslow never put his work on a pyramid, many have taught his theories through this illustration. Self-actualization sits near the top of this chart, right below *transcendence*—a humanistic concept that states we can rise above ourselves to a mystical state where we feel intense joy, peace, and well-being.

Transcendence also asserts that there's a state of personal autonomy—where one can feel completely satisfied in themselves. With all of our needs met, we can become our own gods, dependent on no one. Maslow theorized that we had to have our physical and psychological needs met first, and then we could move on to tapping into our fullest potential as humans.

New Age philosophy builds on these concepts, incorporating spiritual words but directing worship not to the one true God but to the god of self. But Jesus taught something different. His foundation for needs management is to seek first the kingdom of God (Matthew 6:33). **Jesus never said to love ourselves more to find fulfillment; instead, he told us that he is the way, the truth, and the life (John 14:6).**

Your Best Self?

When packaged in a social media meme, self-love and its related principles can *almost* look biblical. "Love yourself first so that you can love others well." Or as one popular author asserts, "Self-love is the fuel that allows an individual to reach their full potential."[1] Messages about becoming our best selves and pouring energy into "loving who we are" have become sprinkled into our Christian music, churches, women's groups, and Bible studies. Some have been paired with an out-of-context Bible verse to lead us away from the gospel of Jesus and toward the false gospel of self.

Jesus didn't model a life of striving for personal betterment. Instead, Jesus's goal was to serve his father and make his kingdom known. His mission was not transcendence—as God, he already had that. Instead, as Philippians 2:7 tells us, Jesus emptied himself so that, even though he was God, he could experience life like we do and model for us how to live.

Pause and read Philippians 2:7. What do you observe about Jesus's life here?

An Upside-Down Kingdom

I recently saw a TikTok of a mom singing in the car while her young daughter sat in the back seat. But it wasn't the alphabet or a *VeggieTales* tune; instead, she crooned a love song to her body. She professed adoration for every part, from nose to toes. The chorus exclaimed something like, "I love how I look!"

Of course, the video had thousands of likes and comments. *What a wonderful message to teach your daughter! Yes! Tell that little girl how to love herself!* But it felt strange to me. My kids learned the Barney song—"I love you, you love me"—which offered a sweet way to bring us all together. But this body-love ballad felt odd, hollow. "I love me, I love me," is a considerably different message from what the purple dinosaur sang.

---

1. Megan Logan, *Self-Love Workbook for Women: Release Self-Doubt, Build Self-Compassion, and Embrace Who You Are* (Emeryville: Rockridge Press, 2020), 3.

Instead of searching for the greatest love of all inside of us, Scripture teaches a better way. The way to find one's life, according to the Bible, is to give it away. The way to be exalted is to be the least. The way to be free is to become a servant to Christ. God's kingdom is upside-down. Jesus didn't come so we could learn to be gods. He came so that we could be reunited with the one true God to spend eternity with him.

It's easy to pick up culture's messages that we need to fill ourselves with self-love or esteem so that we can be free from body image frustration. But filling ourselves is opposite of what Jesus did. The way to be full is to be empty. **We need more of God and less of ourselves.**

In preschool I sang another song, "Jesus Loves Me." The truth in this simple tune cuts through the fluff. When the focus stays on me, it's never enough. But when the focus is on being unconditionally loved by my Maker, I'm free to just be! Self-love isn't the secret to getting comfortable with your reflection; it's humility. Thinking less about who you are and what others think of you and more about who God is and what *he* thinks of you is the best way to find true body image freedom.

Work It Out

Read John 15:13. Who does the Bible point to as the greatest love of all?

Look at 2 Timothy 3:1–3. What does God have to say about self-love?

Do you think self-love is a good thing or a dangerous thing, according to Scripture?

Act

Jesus didn't model striving; he modeled sacrifice. And through his sacrifice, Jesus accomplished the most significant thing in history. While culture teaches that the path to significance is found in striving and getting ahead of others, in Jesus's upside-down kingdom, we feel most significant when we're serving others. Nothing is as effective at getting our minds off our bodies as putting them to work for God's kingdom. Think and pray about some ways you can shift your focus from striving to serving today. Here are some ideas to use as a jumping-off point:

- Show up with a meal for a friend who's going through a busy or challenging season.
- Stop and handwrite a thank-you note to someone who's impacted your life.
- Send three text messages to tell people you are praying for them. (Then pray for them!)
- Offer to run an errand for your spouse, a roommate, or a friend.
- Buy a flower bouquet at the store and surprise a coworker or neighbor.
- Volunteer for a serving role at church.
- Volunteer one hour a month for a local cause you believe in.
- Text your neighbor before you go to the store just to see if they need anything.
- Give a generous tip to someone doing a great job.

Day 32

Trivial Pursuits

Learning not to fear the opinion of others

> If we know God's approval, we won't need to fear any disapproval from others.
>
> *Tim Keller*

"What do you win?"

I ask my client, Hannah, this question and she's quiet. She's just spent ten minutes explaining to me how hard she strives to do everything perfectly. But she's facing a health crisis. She can't keep up. She's still trying to do it all but secretly fears she's letting the people around her down.

So Hannah and I travel back through her past. Trying to do it all, be it all, and please everyone along the way isn't a new pattern. She's followed this program for decades. My question startles her. She stumbles around her emotions to answer, "I guess I feel better?"

With a little humor and a whole lot of grace, I keep her on the hook. "But do you really feel better? Have you ever walked away with the trophy of rest? Have you ever gone to bed thinking, *Okay, I've proven myself, now I can stop trying so hard*?"

Hannah whispers, "No. It's never enough. I'm so tired."

I know exactly what she means. Approval exhausts us.

Who would be disappointed with you if your body never changed in the way you want it to?

Who would you be letting down if you didn't keep working to change your body?

If you were to go away for a year and have your body change significantly, whose opinion of your changed body would you fear? (This answer may reveal whose approval you seek most.)

Elusive Approval

Approval commands us to chase but never lets us catch. It's impossible to have a body that receives approval from everyone in your hemisphere. Neither will your behavior please all the grown-ups all the time. Any actress whose name you know has had her appearance criticized. Models are regularly told they're not thin enough. Some people prefer it when you wear hot pink; others think you should stick to muted tones. **Living for the approval of others is a fast pass for the ride of insecurity.**

Approval always connects to fear. Fear of man. Fear of woman. Fear of my own opinions of myself. *What if I let others down? What if others think I don't look good? What if others think I don't look healthy or don't take care of myself?*

But approval is also about boundaries. *Who is in control of me? Who should have opinions of me? Why am I so influenced by what others think or feel about me?* Poor boundaries connect to body image issues in a variety of ways. Beyond people-pleasing, we find it difficult to follow our own convictions around food, body habits, and even the way we dress. We lack emotional autonomy—we're afraid to make these decisions about ourselves without the input of others. Because others' opinions are vital to how we relate to our bodies, we learn to ignore our body's cues about how we're doing. *If everyone else is smiling and happy, I'm supposed to feel that too. If everyone else is skipping the second slice of pizza, perhaps I shouldn't be hungry either.*

One easy example of this makes me sad to share. There's no need to personalize it because it happens often. A young woman who's gained a few pounds through puberty starts to slim out. Her new figure garners her attention and praise. Well-meaning friends and family members compliment how great she looks. She begins to believe that her slender body size makes her valuable, earning her love and admiration from others. Her identity subtly shifts as she pours new energy into keeping her body small. Soon, an eating disorder is born.

In the early days, she knows skipping meals or working out too hard feels bad for her body. But all the external affirmation inspires her to keep going. *No pain, no gain, right?* She learns that others' opinions of her body are more important than her body's cries for food or rest.

Eventually, the disconnect between what she feels and what others expect of her becomes so great, she learns to separate from her body—mentally and emotionally. Psychologists call it disassociation.

After decades of striving to maintain a certain image, many clients of mine are terrified at the thought that others may not approve of their appearance. Some are still trying to please Mom or Dad (even at age seventy!), while others are still trying to prove to long-gone ex-boyfriends or ex-husbands that their body is good enough to be loved.

They show up at the family graduation or wedding they dreaded, then see the people whose opinions they feared. But even if the responses are positive, it's still not enough. No amount of "Wow, you look great!" compliments can assuage their uncertainty. Even the loudest accolades won't stop their approval-seeking minds from spinning over whether they are truly good enough.

Read Galatians 1:10. What do you learn about people-pleasing from this verse?

Approval Doesn't Lead to Apathy

The call of the gospel is to come as we are. We don't have to polish and perfect ourselves before God approves of us. Through Jesus, I'm already completely accepted. **Nothing will change my relationship status with Jesus.** Fickle family members or fleeting fitness trends won't impact his unflinching approval. **My insecurity melts in his fervent love and grace.**

This doesn't mean I sit on the couch and eat Cheetos all day because I don't care what others think. Instead, a deeper understanding of my acceptance and approval in Christ offers me courageous motivation to live a mentally, physically, and emotionally healthier life. Apathy isn't freedom from approval; it's rebellion. But the one who rebels is still under authority, they've just decided not to listen to it. We're free to live as Jesus has called us to, regardless of what others say or think. That rest my client Hannah longed for? It's found when we live secure in the approval of Christ.

Work It Out

Whose opinion of you matters the most in your heart? Whose approval means the most to you?

What do you hope to win by pleasing yourself or others with the way you look?

In what ways have you confused apathetically not caring about others' opinions with being free to rest in the approval of Jesus?

Are You a People Pleaser? Take This Quiz

☐ I have trouble saying no.

☐ If I do say no, I overexplain the reason why.

☐ I pretend to agree with others so no one gets upset.

☐ I hide my emotions sometimes to protect others.

☐ I tend to act like the people I'm with.

☐ I hate to feel like anyone is mad at me.

☐ I tend to feel responsible for others' emotions
    (if they're upset, it's my fault).

☐ Approval is my oxygen. It's how I know I'm okay.

☐ Nothing feels better than when people praise me.

☐ I apologize a lot, maybe too much.

If you have three or more check marks, it may be time to evaluate your people-pleasing tendencies.

ABC's for People Pleasers

Adopt a new motto: "God is the only one I have to please."

Build better boundaries. You are allowed to make your own decisions. Begin to recognize people in your life who always want you to conform to their way, and pray for God to give you the courage to say no when you need to.

Choose who you are responsible for and who you are responsible to. You do not have to answer for everyone; nor do you have to answer *to* everyone.

Day 33

Don't Believe Everything You Think

Retiring from mental gymnastics

> I was trapped in a battle that took place 24/7, and it . . . began to defeat me.
> My mirror, my pictures, my clothes, and my view were my worst enemies.
>
> *Sadie Robertson Huff*

There are both physical and psychological factors at work that keep us believing, doing, and thinking the same things over and over again. Neuroplasticity explains how our brains adapt to information. This is how our brains stay organized after repeatedly practicing an activity or processing a memory. Neurons fire up and, as scientists explain, get wired together. The more times you make this electric connection, the easier it is to make that association over again. If you've learned not to touch a cookie sheet straight from the oven, thank your brain for helping you stay comfortable and pain-free.

But what if the things you've taught your brain simply aren't true? What if you've convinced your brain that your body is unacceptable or that it's unsafe to wear a certain size? What if every time you eat something sweet, your brain signals feelings of guilt? What if those well-worn neural pathways seem to re-emphasize just how unlovable, unacceptable, or undesirable you are because of your body? Is there hope?

The short answer is *yes*.

Changing Your Brain

Our brains are more malleable than once understood. Even though messages shout from all around us, we *can* learn to change those neuropathways and calm the war that wages between our ears. Now I can take thoughts captive and speak back to my brain when I become overfocused on a perceived body flaw. Changing neuropathways takes time. If you've been working your way through this book, there's a good chance you're already starting to feel the thought patterns change. Now is the push to engrave new patterns and thoughts.

What thought patterns do you feel like you still need to change in your life?

Taking Thoughts to Court

1) **The Thought:** Write it or speak it.

2) **The Defense:** Write out any evidence you can think of that defends the thought.

3) **The Prosecution:** Write out any evidence you can think of that refutes the thought.
   Pro Tip → Read what Scripture says about your thoughts.

4) **The Judge's Verdict:** Is the original thought accurate and fair?

In a trial, evidence can only be used if it's a verifiable FACT. No interpretation, guesses, or opinions.

Thanks to Brittany Braswell, RD, for this exercise.

You Don't Have to Believe Everything You Think

Here's a great reminder: **If having a great body led to having a great relationship, Hollywood would be the mecca of happy marriages.** But it's not. In fact, those who've reached elite status in the realm of physical appearance may have even more relational struggles than the rest of us. But the lie that *If I looked better, my marriage would be better* (or *I'd have a man*) bounces around, pretending to be an encyclopedia fact. *It's not.*

Philippians 4:8 offers helpful instructions for our thought lives. It reads like this, "And now, dear brothers and sisters, one final thing. Fix your thoughts on what is true, and honorable, and right, and pure, and lovely, and admirable. Think about things that are excellent and worthy of praise" (NLT).

When we're thinking about how awful it is that our bellies pooch or our hair is thinning, are we thinking thoughts about our body that are right, pure, lovely, and admirable? When we believe we'd have a better sex life if we had a more sculpted physique, we're not meditating on what is true or right.

Romans 12:2 gives us the wisdom we need to support changing our neural pathways: "Do not conform to the pattern of this world, but be transformed by the renewing of your mind. Then you will be able to test and approve what God's will is—his good, pleasing and perfect will."

Renewing our minds means thinking differently in order to change those well-worn pathways of defeating, negative, or untrue thoughts about ourselves and our bodies. This isn't a one-and-done act where we hit our heads and suddenly see ourselves as gorgeous—like in the movie *I Feel Pretty*. It's a process. The word translated as *transformed* comes from the same root as *metamorphosis*. The change isn't partial or indistinguishable. The work is a total transformation.[1]

The result of renewing your mind is better than any makeover. **Consider this: When we desire body change, isn't rest what we really crave?** We long for the freedom to stop obsessing, and we believe changing our bodies will grant that, but it doesn't. Only the renewing of our mind can have this impact.

---

1. David Guzik, "Romans 12—Living the Christian Life," Enduring Word, December 23, 2015, https://enduring word.com/bible-commentary/romans-12/.

We don't have to believe everything we think. It takes faith to understand that God's thoughts are not just higher than ours, but they're also more accurate! (See Isaiah 55:8–9.) Who am I to believe that my own opinions of me are truer than those of the Almighty?

Look up Isaiah 55:8–9. Can you believe that it's more important to believe God's thoughts about your body than your own?

The Living Sacrifice

This same passage in Romans 12 ends with our brains but starts with our bodies. Verse 1 instructs us to make our bodies a living sacrifice. Paul makes a radical statement here because Jews were only familiar with sacrifices that involved dead animals. But a living sacrifice would stay alive, on the altar indefinitely. We don't have to go slay an animal (*thank God!*), but I do have to lay down my desire to control all the things all the time. *Hmm . . . maybe the sheep thing would be easier.* In fact, Paul urges his readers that true and proper worship starts with letting go of the one thing that, if you're reading this book, you may hesitate to surrender—your body!

Surrendering our body image means accepting that God's standards and truth rule. When we struggle with image, there are often other standards ruling the way we measure ourselves. We've conformed to the pressures of this world (Romans 12:2). The exercise below can help you identify how you're measuring yourself and help you reframe your thinking to use God's measurement standards.

Work It Out

Grab an inexpensive ruler and meditate on these questions as you hold that ruler in your hand. Watch the video at improvebodyimage.com/ruler-exercise that explains the exercise. Then journal your answers to these questions.

What standard do I use to measure my value and worth? How do I compare myself to others using this standard?

Why should I live by this standard of measure?

Does anyone else in my life measure me this way?

Who is the true ruler of my life? God and his standards or the standard of my ruler?

Read James 4. What does this teach us about "God's ruler"—how does he measure us? What does he hate? What does he love?

Put your ruler somewhere you will see it daily to be reminded of how free you are from these earthly ways of measuring yourself.

Day 34

You're a Masterpiece

But it's not about the art

For we are God's masterpiece. He has created us anew in Christ Jesus, so
we can do the good things he planned for us long ago.

Ephesians 2:10 NLT

Perhaps you've heard that you're God's masterpiece. You've read the verse or
gone to a church women's event where the topic of body image came up. Perhaps
the speaker made you shout it. "I'm God's masterpiece!"

If you're like me, remembering this biblical truth helped for a few minutes or
hours. But as soon as the meeting broke for lunch, I was right back to comparing myself to others. *If we're all masterpieces, I'm not that special.* And wasn't it
possible that some of the masterpieces were main-gallery floor quality, while
my kind of masterpiece belonged in the museum basement?

I'd let culture's definitions of beauty and success replace God's definition
of a masterpiece.

What is your definition of a masterpiece?

Masterpiece Theater

Masterpiece defines a special, unique, or exquisite creation. But we often forget that the work of art isn't inherently good. To be qualified as a masterpiece requires the intelligence, skill, workmanship, and ingenuity of a master.

When Scripture tells us that we are God's masterpiece, it's not a command to love the way we look. Instead, it's to remind us *who* it is that formed, shaped, and designed us, and *who* continues to mold and sanctify us.

If I worship the masterpiece apart from the master, I have no objective source to judge its merit. If Rembrandt painted it or Michelangelo sculpted it, museums don't overanalyze what it looks like—they just want it in their collection. But my daughter's preschool paintings, though a great treasure to me because I love the artist, will not sell for millions at auction. The beauty of art is subjective apart from knowledge of the artist.

How should remembering who created you remind you of your value?

In Romans 9, Paul tells the church that they are God's handiwork and that God gets to choose how he uses them. In a powerful word picture, Paul talks about jars of clay. He asks his audience if the clay can tell the potter how to form it. Of course the clay can't. Neither would the clay tell the potter that he was doing a terrible job or, worse, had done it "wrong." Paul encourages us not to question God's ways, reminding us that he is the potter and we are the clay. In other words, he's painting the Mona Lisa on our lives. Are we like kindergarteners with crayons, thinking we can improve the picture?

No one wants to remain an unformed vessel—a "before" picture. So one question lies before us daily. **Will we continue to be formed by the potter into the vessel he desires us to be? Or will we be deformed by the culture into the type of beauty or person that we believe we need to be so we can feel accepted in this kingdom?**

Respond to the questions above. Give words to how you feel your formation process is going.

The Masterpiece Principle

Considering yourself a masterpiece isn't about body pride. It's about tilting your mirror up to recognize your most important work here is to reflect the artist. This takes the pressure off. You don't have to look perfect. You simply have to reflect the One in whose image you were made. The real beauty that the master is crafting is in your heart. **While we strive to make the outside of our earthly houses look better, God wants to transform our lives from the inside out.**

First Peter 3:3–4 discusses how our true beauty shouldn't come from our physical beauty but from a gentle and quiet spirit. This passage always bothered me, though. I'm a talker. Sometimes I'm too loud. It felt like this was just one more standard I was failing. *Add it to the list.*

But now I know that a gentle and quiet spirit isn't about being a people pleaser. Instead, a gentle and quiet spirit is one that exudes peace. She's the woman who walks into the room and sees other people instead of wondering if they see her. She's gentle because she's put aside the harsh ways the world teaches us to relate to one another and, instead, she's content to cultivate her inner beauty. She's quiet, not because she doesn't have opinions, but because she can rest from the mental gymnastics of what it takes to be noticed.

As God's masterpiece, you're free from the burden of trying to prove your body is good enough. You can trust God to help you let the beauty of your heart shine through so that all can see your true beauty. Let Jesus speak peace to the storm inside your brain when you believe the lies that you're not acceptable.

Work It Out

What would it look like to live like you're already a masterpiece, free from the pressure to tweak or perfect yourself culture's way?

Now, allow yourself to dream a bit. How would you feel after a full year of walking in the freedom to reflect God's beauty, without the pressure to imitate what culture deems beautiful?

What does a "gentle and quiet spirit" mean to you?

Act

Grab a handheld mirror and then watch the mirror tilt exercise video at improvebodyimage.com/mirror-tilt/.

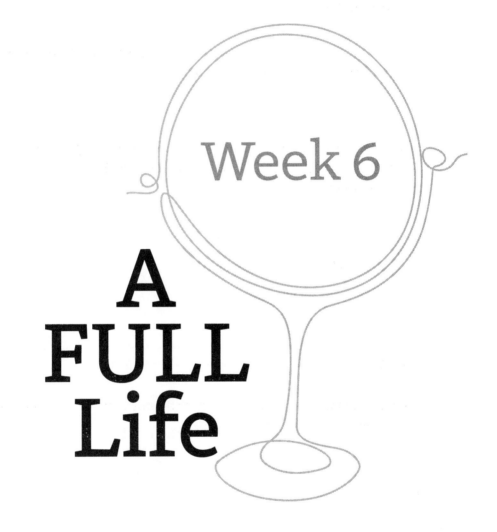

Week 6

A FULL Life

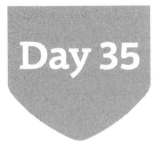

Day 35

Thanking God for Your Body

How gratitude changes your attitude

Yes, give thanks for "all things" for, as it has been well said, "Our disappointments are but His appointments."

A. W. Pink

Sometimes God asks us to do things we'd rather not. Years after I published my first book and recorded numerous podcast episodes on the topic of body image, God convicted me that I was still missing it. While sitting in a circle with a few other leaders from our church, reading and praying through Psalm 16, I felt God clearly say, "Heather, thank me for your body."

Hmm . . . thank you for my body? Interesting concept, Lord. You've done so much to help me accept it. But thank you for it? That kind of feels like you want me to say I like my body. I'm not sure I'm ready for—

"Heather, thank me for your body."

I'm learning that when God asks, I need to obey. So I did. Out loud, in front of male and female witnesses, I thanked God for my body. It was clunky. It was awkward. No, I take that back. It was just weird.

But the verse that stuck out to me was from Psalm 16:6. In some translations, including the NIV, it reads, "The boundary lines have fallen for me in pleasant places." That day, I read it as my silhouette. My lot, my inheritance, my portion—these words all spoke clearly to my body, my weight, my genetics, and my build—how much space I take up on the planet. **Could I believe these boundaries God had set for my physical body were pleasant?** Could I trust that it was okay to take up space? *On that day I did.*

Grateful for Cellulite?

One aspect of the body positivity movement that has always struck me as strange is this concept of loving those parts of our body that no one actually likes. It feels so disingenuous. *Really? You love the look of cellulite?*

So where's the line between accepting your body and being an exhibitionist? What's the difference between being thankful for your body and body love? It all comes down to thanking God even when we can't understand the what or the why; we acknowledge he's in charge, no matter what. Some call that trust.

God is gracious. As we begin a journey toward being thankful for our bodies, he is patient with us. There are parts of my body I was able to thank him for immediately. I could thank him that my body carried each of my four babies. I could thank him that my hair doesn't offend me most days. I could thank him that my feet look pretty when my toenails are painted.

Start slow. God doesn't ask you to write your body a sonnet. That's the advice of culture. Frankly, I don't know if I'll ever be able to love everything I see in the mirror—especially without clothes on! Biblically, loving our bodies means respecting and caring for them as God's good creation, while culturally, "body love" often means body pride. Real love, we know from 1 Corinthians 13:5, is never self-seeking or self-focused.

But with each passing day, the more grateful I am, the more my heart softens. I sense my body's purpose. I see God's good creation. I appreciate how my body keeps me safe, allows me to show up in the world, and digests dark chocolate without giving me acid reflux. *At least most of the time.*

Gradually, my tight grip on body control and my expectations for my size or appearance loosen. It doesn't happen all at once, but you may be surprised when you first start to feel the shift. **The desire to have a better body is much like desiring more wealth.** If you fixate on it, chase it, and put all your energy into getting rich, you'll never be satisfied. But once you start to count your blessings, you find that what you have is always enough.

Gratefulness doesn't start with loving your body. It starts with accepting that God has a bigger purpose for me than looking good in a bikini. And science backs it up. Higher levels of gratitude connect to lower levels of body shame.[1]

Eyes Up

Remember: Acknowledging the giver's heart is more important than liking the gift.

As we mature, we learn that gifts are a bond between giver and recipient. I enjoy the gift, but it is the giver's kindness or thoughtfulness that touches my heart. When we tell God we are grateful for our bodies, the focus shouldn't be on our opinion of his gift. **Our gratitude can center on our opinion of the Giver.**

I trust God is a good Father. Therefore, I can thank him, confidently acknowledging that if he thought this body was good for me—then it is! Do I fantasize that life would be better if I were taller, tanner, and tighter? *Sometimes.* But when I snap back to reality, I remember that God didn't create me to go on display. He wants me to use this gift to serve and worship him.

Why'd God give me thick thighs and short fingers? I don't know. Add it to the list of God's mysteries. His ways are not my ways (Isaiah 55:8–9). I can trust that he knew what he was doing and be thankful, even if I never figure out the why.

Beware of Comparison

Nothing kills gratitude like comparison. Perhaps you've experienced it too. I can feel comfortable in my home until I spend a few hours watching HGTV. Suddenly, everything around me looks outdated. I convince myself we should never have guests over. We obviously need a home makeover.

The same is true for my body. As my gratitude grows for the gift of my body, I can start to feel at home in it. Until I'm exposed to images of "better houses." Then my gratitude fades. I wonder how I can ever go out in public again until I "fix" all that's wrong with my earthly dwelling.

---

1. Alisha M. Wenger, "The Impact of Gratitude on Body Image, Exercise, and Eating Behaviors," (PsyD, diss., George Fox University, 2020), iii, https://digitalcommons.georgefox.edu/cgi/viewcontent.cgi?article=1344&context=psyd.

The more we compare, the more we despair. Comparison kills contentment, while gratitude grows it. Kicking the comparison habit is vital to having healthy and holy feelings about your body. (Just so happens I wrote a whole book on this topic. If this is a struggle for you, go check it out.)

Work It Out

Is it easy or difficult for you to thank the Giver for his gift of your body?

When do you find it easier to be grateful for your body? Are there certain times when it is more difficult to thank God for your body?

What can you be thankful for today, as it relates to your body? Time yourself for two minutes and write down as many things as you can think of. You can start by being grateful for opposable thumbs and a beating heart. God will meet you where you're at, if that's all the further you get today. But I bet you can think of several ways you are specifically grateful for your body.

My Gratefulness List

Act

Prayer of Gratitude

Use your gratefulness list and write a prayer thanking God for your body.

Dear Heavenly Father, thank you for my body.

_____

_____

_____

_____

_____

_____

Day 36

Living the FULL Life

Focused above and unconditionally loved

> The purposes of a person's heart are deep waters, but one who has insight draws them out.
>
> *Proverbs 20:5*

I've sung "I surrender all" to God, hands raised, while simultaneously wondering what the people worshiping around me thought of my outfit. *There, I said it.*

I flash back to my youth group days when I feared God would make me become a missionary to Africa. *But I can't survive without air conditioning, Lord!* What if I surrender my body to God, but his idea of how my body should look isn't the same as mine? What if he *wants* me to look bad? Perhaps the question is: Can God *really* be trusted to do what I think he should do with my body? *Yikes! What if I never like the way I look in pictures?*

It's subtle, but the fear is genuine. **I'm happy to surrender to God's will in other areas of my life. But does Scripture really tell me that God gets to decide what happens with my body?** Perhaps, since there aren't clear instructions on what we should weigh or how we should style our hair, maybe I *can* be in control of that?

There's a story in Matthew 22 where the Pharisees are trying to trap Jesus into saying something that could get him arrested. The topic: paying taxes. Jesus outsmarts them, of course, and directs them to look at a Roman coin. Whose *image* is on the coin, Jesus asks. There's no confusion there. So Jesus easily responds, "Give to Caesar what belongs to Caesar, and give to God what belongs to God" (Matthew 22:21 NLT).

You may be wondering how this connects to our body image issues. But follow me here. If we are God's image bearers, whose image is on us? God's, right? So who are our bodies for? Who do we surrender our image to? Who should be most pleased with our bodies and what we do with them? My friends, my family, myself . . . or the One whose image I bear? **Could the secret to solving our body image issues be as simple as surrendering to God what is already his?**

How does the thought of surrendering your appearance to God make you feel? What thoughts or concerns come to mind?

A New Job

Many of my clients have also felt the shift from full-time body change fixation to mental freedom. Some remark, "I'm not sure what to do now that I don't spend all my time thinking about my body!" It may be uncomfortable at first to get that mental space back. You may feel like you *should* be stressing about your body, as if that was the "responsible" thing to do. But remember, *should* is black-and-white thinking. You're living in the grace to steward your body well without making it an obsession. You can live free!

So what do you do if you're not on a full-time quest to fix your body? You live a FULL life. FULL is an acronym that stands for

> Focused above,
>
> Unconditionally loved,
>
> Living in freedom, and
>
> Living in fullness.

Over the next few days, we'll examine each aspect of this kind of living.

Focused Above

Body image issues are like a bug on your windshield. If you focus on the bug, everything else in your view will get fuzzy. But if you focus on the bigger picture, you'll barely notice that little bug. Maybe a better example is your scale.

If you focus on that one number on that one little box, you miss out on seeing the enormity of life all around you.

As Christ followers, we're called to keep our focus somewhere specific—on Jesus. We're encouraged to fix our thoughts on things that are above (Colossians 3:2). Here are some practical ways to keep your heart and gaze focused above every day.

> **Read your Bible every day.** If this is a new practice to you, start with You-Version, the Bible app, and read passages connected to one of my reading plans. Read the verse of the day, and as you can, read the chapter it comes from. Time spent reading God's Word is never wasted and will always encourage you and ground you in the truth. If you want to define beauty the way the Word does, you have to be reminded of this as frequently as you're reminded of the world's definition (2 Timothy 3:16).

> **Pray without ceasing.** Ask the Holy Spirit, the Counselor, to help you through these struggles. Invite him to show you where you're stuck, to convict you of idols and sin, and to help you navigate food issues. Pray specifically for God to help you stop comparing yourself to other women, to help you stop defining beauty the world's way, and to help you see yourself the way he does. Though we may have convinced ourselves that God doesn't want to hear it when we feel uncomfortable in our bodies, this is unhelpful. We are God's precious children. He wants us to come to him so he can remind us of his love (1 Thessalonians 5:17–19).

> **Be in Christian community.** The Bible instructs us to be in community with other believers. If your only friends are unbelievers or your only community is at the gym, it will be harder to remember that God has a purpose for your life beyond improving your body (Hebrews 10:25).

Unconditionally Loved

The enemy will take every opportunity he can to make you feel unloved and unsafe unless you focus on "fixing" your body. Hopefully, now you understand that these are lies to be fought, not truths to live by. Here are a few ideas of ways to remind yourself of God's great love for you.

- Create a screen saver with your favorite verse about God's love. Put it on your phone or computer's lock screen so you read it several times a day.
- Write the words "You are Unconditionally Loved and Accepted by the God of the Universe" on the top of your mirror.
- Put a sticky note on your scale's readout that says, "You are already loved," that you must peel off before you weigh yourself. You may need to put multiple notes with verses or other biblical encouragement so you can read several before you see that number. (Note: Most of us are probably better off without that scale's judgment, but if you're not there yet, do this!)
- Wear a cross necklace or carry something that reminds you of God's love for you in your pocket. When you feel afraid, insecure, or uncertain, you can feel it.
- Research and study God's love for you. Reference these verses: John 3:16; 1 John 4:9–11; 1 John 4:16; Romans 8:37–39; Romans 5:8.

Work It Out

I know God loves me because . . .

God's love changes the way I see my body because . . .

God's love gives me security, approval, and rest because . . .

Day 37

Living in Freedom

Habits that keep you free

> It is for freedom that Christ has set us free. Stand firm, then, and do not let yourselves be burdened again by a yoke of slavery.
>
> *Galatians 5:1*

As a single woman in her twenties, Gladys Aylward traveled to China to tell people about Jesus. What she didn't expect was how God would also use her to unbind their feet.

Foot binding had been a tradition for Chinese women for more than a thousand years. Between the ages of five and eight, a girl would have her feet wrapped so that the four smaller toes would bend toward the bottom of her foot. In this position, the foot would develop a distinct arch and be restricted from further growth. Girls faced infections of all kinds—including gangrene—and often lost toes in the process. The goal was for women to have feet that were no longer than four inches. Reaching "Golden Lotus" status meant not only that your feet were the perfect shape, but that you were among the most attractive, erotic, and elegant. Girls had to be taught to walk in a different way, and the pain was often intolerable.[1]

Cartwright explains that though the trend began among dancers and others in more promiscuous occupations, the trend caught on in the upper classes, and the practice connected to their worship of a Buddhist idol—Guanyin—who

---

1. Mark Cartwright, "Foot-Binding," World History Encyclopedia, September 27, 2017, https://www.worldhistory.org/Foot-Binding/.

was thought to protect women.[2] For hundreds of years, foot binding symbolized submission, beauty, and worship.

Though there had been previous attempts to ban the practice, it wasn't until 1912 that new laws were put in place to prohibit this destructive trend. When Gladys arrived in the country in 1930, she was hired by the Chinese government as a foot inspector to tour the country to make sure that mothers and grandmothers were no longer binding their daughters' feet. But for Gladys, this was an opportunity to free women not only from the bondage of broken and crippled toes, but from the bondage of slavery to sin. In Isaiah 52:7 we read, "How beautiful . . . are the feet of those who bring good news." I bet Gladys Aylward's feet were the most beautiful these women had ever seen.

Freedom from Rituals That Bind Us

Did you notice that foot binding started as a practice of women in sex-related industries and gradually spread throughout all of Chinese society? How many of our body ideals are influenced by the sex industry today? There's no doubt that our definitions of beauty have been distorted by pornography of all types. Our hyper-sexualized culture teaches us that unless your body is lust-worthy, you're not loveable. **To walk in freedom, we must recognize that many of our culture's beauty expectations are crippling to the ones trying to uphold them.** From eating disorders and overexercising to surgical procedures to get the perfect selfie, maybe culturally we're not all that different from those who bound their feet to be beautiful. Living in freedom means untethering ourselves from culture's definitions and beauty standards.

Living in Freedom Takes Intentionality

Living in freedom doesn't mean you'll never have a negative thought about your body again. Neither does it mean that tomorrow you'll wake up and not care about your clothes, your weight, or complexion.

Instead, freedom means that you no longer obsess over these things. Freedom looks like having coping mechanisms to know how to fight, and having a

---

2. Cartwright, "Foot-Binding."

plan for what to do when the spiral starts. When you're on the freedom path, you begin to feel increasingly comfortable in your body as it is. Sometimes you may fantasize about the ideal you or be tempted to Google "How to lose 10 pounds in 3 days," but you will remember that *that* path never led to anything healthy. Here are some other strategies to continue living in freedom:

- **Keep this book and re-read your answers periodically.** This will remind you of how far you've come, especially when you have a bad body image day and Satan tells you that you've made no progress at all.

- **Connect with God.** As you feel yourself drawn to serving image, beauty, or other idols, you may feel like God's love for you fades. It doesn't! But to feel reconnected with him, stop, confess, repent, and ask him to help you feel his love covering you.

- **Worship.** Worship is the best way to cure bad body image days. When you're feeling low, turn to worship. Blare your favorite worship tunes and sing along, turning your attention from your body and these "momentary afflictions" (2 Corinthians 4:17 ESV) and back to God. I've found that raising my hands is a physical way of surrendering my body—and body image—to God and allowing him to show me that he is the one worthy of worship, not me. Praise is the culmination of our delight. When we love something or someone, we want to tell the world about it! Like leaving a five-star review for that new restaurant you love, public praise fulfills our delight (Psalm 66).

- **Rest.** Everything goes haywire when you're not sleeping well. Autopilot switches on, and we tend to go back to our addictions and coping mechanisms ("What's my next diet?"). Recognize your need for rest and prioritize it. Similarly, recognize that if you feel body image issues flaring, you may be overtired.

- **Don't be afraid to face your emotions.** Being honest about your emotions related to your body and appearance is key to staying free. When you feel discouraged, alone, or hopeless, find a trusted friend or a counselor you can talk to in these seasons. Remember that God is always there to listen and comfort you too. Taking the time to identify and deal with emotions as they arise will help you continue to walk in freedom.

- **Be patient with those who don't understand** your journey. Your husband, boyfriend, or best friends may all be confused as to why you no longer want to fixate on changing your body. You may be accused of being "unhealthy" or worse. You may try to explain that body image issues became an obstacle to your mental health. But know that not everyone will understand. If you feel alone, seek encouragement and help from a professional to stay the course. Your freedom is worth it.

Work It Out

What or who has most influenced your body ideals? What would it feel like to be untethered from your personal definitions of beauty in order to embrace God's?

What are two strategies from above (or your own) that you can commit to in order to intentionally keep walking in freedom?

Living in Fullness

Keeping a healthy perspective

> Why are we thinking so much about what we physically look like? That's the biggest trick that's ever been played on women. If we're so preoccupied with our looks, we'll never develop any of our talents.
>
> *Christina Ricci*

I seem to gain several pounds every time I write a book. I'm not sure if it's the extra sitting or the chocolate I consume when I can't find the right words. This is book number four, so if you do the math, you'll see the depths of my sacrifice. As a woman who's battled the scale her whole life, some days I still struggle to believe that my greatest contribution to the world isn't related to shrinking my body.

I've gotten better at brushing that false belief aside, though, even on days when my jeans don't fit. Writing books makes me feel alive in ways that being "thinner" never could. The buzz of hitting a goal weight is nothing compared to the joy of hearing how you've helped someone draw closer to God and his purpose for their life. As Luke 12:23 reminds us, life is so much more than food. Our bodies are more than just mannequins to display clothing.

This is the full life! When you know why you were made and who you were created to worship, you aren't emotionally or mentally held back by what you believe about the appearance of your body. You feel God's purpose pulsing through your veins. You're ready to serve and no longer afraid of what others

think. You know that God's opinion of your body is more important than theirs
... and your own!

Here are some ways to practice living a full life:

Don't be afraid of being full. Do whatever it takes to get into a healthy relationship with food where you can eat enough to fuel your body, feel satisfied,
and overcome destructive behaviors like restricting and bingeing. For years I
tried not to eat anything until lunchtime. Every day I felt exhausted by 1 p.m.,
and most days, I needed an afternoon nap to function. A strange thing happened when I started eating breakfast. I actually had more energy all day long
and could use my former nap time to take a walk or get work done. Remember:
Food is not the enemy. (Neither is it a suitable best friend.) If you need support
in this area, use the link from the Need More Help? section at the back of this
book to find someone to gently guide you to food freedom.

Move when and how you need to. Exercise can help you feel better about your
body, physically and mentally. Choose types of movement that feel comfortable
and enjoyable to you. If you hate running, don't sign up for a marathon just so
you can get the 26.2 bumper sticker. If step aerobics almost landed you in the
hospital (*maybe that's just me*), choose workouts that don't require excellent
coordination. The best type of exercise for your health isn't the one that's most
popular. It's the one you enjoy and will do regularly because you like it!

Watch what you watch. Psalm 119:37 (ESV) instructs, "Turn my eyes from
looking at worthless things; and give me life in your ways." If you're constantly
looking at images, ads, articles, and other visuals that remind you of the world's
definition of beauty and value, you'll feel the life sap away from your bones. Do
you know that pitted feeling you get after scrolling social media or watching
certain shows? Looking at unhealthy things can literally give us a stomachache.
Listen to that gut feeling—turn off the screen, turn to God's Word, and worship.
Build yourself up in his truth. A media diet is the only rigid diet I'll ever endorse.
It's time to get strict about what you look at!

Wear clothing that makes you feel alive. It doesn't have to be expensive, but
clothing that fits you well will help you feel better in your body and will keep you
free to think about living and enjoying life! It's hard to focus on loving others
when your Spanx are suffocating. I've noticed that a too-tight waistband makes

it nearly impossible for me to tell if I'm hungry or full, which also impacts my relationship with food. Have some go-to wardrobe items that feel comfortable and that you feel confident wearing on those bad body image days when you're afraid of everything else in your closet. Remember, clothes were intended to fit the body, not the other way around.

Find other things that you enjoy doing. Body change is not a hobby. Hobbies are activities that help you relax and have fun. Do you have some? If not, it's time to try a few things you've always considered but maybe never had the confidence or time to pursue. Take an art class, try pickleball, or learn to cook. See how alive you feel when you find something you enjoy.

Serve. If you can rattle off what you ate today faster than you can list your spiritual gifts, it's time to figure out how God wired you. Take a free spiritual-gifts test online and then try to find areas in your church or community where you can use them! You'll be surprised at how alive, embodied, and free you feel when you're using your God-given gifts!

From the FULL list above, what are three things you can work on incorporating into your life this week? Write them here and then ask a friend to keep you accountable to trying them:

1. _____

   _____

2. _____

   _____

3. _____

   _____

My Spiritual Gifts Are:

Work It Out

What is one thing you'd like to accomplish this month that is unrelated to your body?

What is one thing you'd like to accomplish this year that is unrelated to your body?

What to Do on a Bad Body Image Day

If you wake up feeling lousy about your body, don't get on the scale or look to the mirror to cheer you up. Instead, do this:

1) Ask: What am I thinking about? Remind yourself of Philippians 4:8 and run your thoughts through that filter.
2) Ask: Am I stressed about something else but projecting that stress onto my body? Will changing or trying to control my body fix what I'm stressed about?
3) Ask: Is anyone as focused on the way my body looks today as I am?
4) Ask: What am I believing will rescue me from the emotional discomfort I feel right now? Am I turning to Jesus, or am I believing that a different body would bring me the joy, peace, and rest that only Jesus can?

Day 39

Soli Deo Gloria

Remembering where the glory goes

> Humility is nothing but the disappearance of self in the vision that God is all.
>
> *Andrew Murray*

It's hard for our human brains to imagine heaven. Gold-covered streets and *all* that singing? Sometimes it sounds a little odd. But I can't wait! *Why?* Because, among other reasons, I'll finally be completely free of body image issues.

They won't disappear because my heavenly body will be the perfect size or shape—though I'm pretty sure I've heard a portly pastor teach it that way. **Rather, in heaven it'll be clear who deserves all the glory.** My desire to have any glory for myself will disappear, and the pressure to be glory-worthy will be completely removed. In Latin, the phrase is *Soli Deo gloria*—all the glory goes to God. If only I could remember that here on earth. My job is not to garner glory but to reflect his.

The Oldest Struggle in the Book

You may remember that Satan, the devil, whatever you prefer to call him, wasn't always opposed to God. He was once a guardian cherub, the most beautiful of all the angels. But, according to Ezekiel 28:11–19, his heart became proud because of his own beauty and desire for glory. Scripture tells us that we are now engaged in spiritual warfare, every day. **And it all started over Satan's pride. He decided he was so hot, he didn't need God.** Every time I'm tempted to believe that more beauty will solve my body image issues, I wonder, *What if more beauty would just make them worse?*

We may *ooh* and *ahh* over how "good" someone looks in their casket (*and isn't it weird that we get all dolled up to be buried? Sigh*), but our bodies are not our legacies. My weight won't be engraved on my headstone (*praise God!*). Even if someday my grandchildren look at a picture and decide Grandma was beautiful, they'll still think I dressed like an old person and wore a strange hairstyle.

Romans 11:36 (NLT) reminds us, "For everything comes from him and exists by his power and is intended for his glory. All glory to him forever!" If I can just remember where the glory goes, my body image issues fade. If I can keep my eyes fixed up at my Savior instead of down at my stomach, how much freer will I feel?

Likewise, even in those times when I do get attention—if friends comment that I look nice, or a stranger gives me a second glance—what would it be like to bounce the glory back to God? I work with many women who wrestle body image issues while, simultaneously, receiving a lot of attention for their physical appearance. Their temptation is to feed on the compliments, then obsess over "what's wrong" on days they don't get them. We work together to practice directing body praise right back to the source of our glory. They practice saying things like *Soli Deo gloria* to deflect praise back to the one whom we image: God.

Work It Out

Getting ready for church was a battlefield for me for many years. I wanted to look "good" enough for others to notice me. One day I realized that, subtly, I desired a little of God's glory—even in the place designed to worship him! Have you done this? *In what ways have you wrestled the desire to have "some" glory for yourself?*

Act

If you have negative body thoughts this week, or as you receive compliments or praise for your appearance, practice speaking these words to yourself in English or in Latin! Soli Deo gloria, *or All glory to God!*

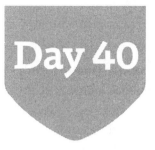

Day 40

Be Like Moses

Don't go back to Egypt

> Do not love the world or the things in the world. If anyone loves the world, the love of the Father is not in him.
>
> *1 John 2:15 ESV*

We started this journey with the story of an old guy from Genesis. Let's end it with the story of another old guy from Exodus: Moses.

Poor Moses. He certainly had his hands full. After carting four young children through Costco and Target, I learned to hate that expression. But it may be apt for old Mo's situation. He led the people out of bondage, out of slavery. They were headed to a promised land, and what did they do? They asked if they could go back to Egypt. *Sigh.*

I pray this book has opened your eyes to a new way of thinking about your body and body image. I hope you're ready to walk free from the tyranny of diet culture and the oppressive thoughts about your body that have held you captive. I want you to taste the freedom of a life that isn't spent obsessing over your body. But let me just be straight with you. **There will come a day when you'll want to go back to Egypt because you'll believe life was somehow better in the prison of body image bondage.**

- Your friend will lose a bazillion pounds on her new starvation diet, and you'll sign up for the program.

- Your mom will forget to tell you that you look nice on Easter, and you'll spiral into fear over what she thinks of you and your body.
- Your husband will stare a little too long at the cheerleaders on the screen, and you'll Google liposuction and Botox.
- You'll see a picture of yourself and determine you should burn that outfit and never leave the house again. (Reference Day 9!)
- The doctor's office scales, the dressing room mirror, and your favorite jeans will band together to tell you that you're unlovable all on the same day.

This is reality, my friend. You can't escape diet culture unless you move to an island without internet connection. Jesus said we should be in the world but not of it (John 15:19; 17:14–16). The call to love what the world loves, worship beauty like the world worships it, and seek rescue the way everyone else does blares like your neighbor's car alarm triggered in a thunderstorm.

So how can we keep walking toward freedom? How can we remember to seek the Savior—not the scale—for salvation from our shame? Here are some final ideas.

Don't go back to Egypt. Don't go back to the way you've always done things. Have faith that God is growing you and working in your life to change you from the inside out. Stay diligent with all you've learned here, and give the Holy Spirit space to walk with you on this new path away from the world's ways of "fixing" your body image issues.

Read Isaiah 31. What does it mean to seek help from the Lord as you continue this journey?

Make your own support group. If you feel alone in this new way of thinking about body image issues, create your own support group. Chances are, most of the women you know struggle in some way with these same challenges. Invite them to read and go through the content of this book with you. Invite them to listen to my podcast, *Compared to Who?*, with you. It's a podcast where I offer weekly encouragement, biblical truth, and practical strategies to help you fight and win your battles with insecurity, body shame, comparison, and approval. The best way to learn may be to teach. We grow when we take bold steps of faith. Even if you don't feel like a natural leader, simply inviting a few friends to hang out and talk about it once a week is a great way to keep you on the right track while encouraging others.

Who are two or three women in your life right now who may need some encouragement in the body image arena?

Who would you like to read and discuss this book with?

Sing a new song to the Lord. Isaiah 42:10 tells us to sing a new song to the Lord. Thank God for what he's done in your life and acknowledge what's new— what's new in your thinking, your attitude, your perspective, your habits. *Write these down.*

That old song—the soundtrack you've blared in your brain for years, decades, forever—may come back. It may play loud. I once crooned, "Oh, God, just make me skinny." But my new song is, "God, help me use my body to honor you." You too can sing a new song. It will feel awkward, uncomfortable, and unfamiliar. Change and growth are always worth it.

Read Isaiah 42:10. If you were to write the lyrics for your new song, how would they read?

Be open to God doing a new thing. In Isaiah 43:19 (ESV), we read, "Behold, I am doing a new thing; now it springs forth, do you not perceive it? I will make a way in the wilderness and rivers in the desert." Friend, you have nothing to be afraid of on this journey! Getting "thinner," "healthier," or "better looking" will not change how the Father loves you. He wants you, as you are today, to come to him with open hands and ask him for help. **Trust him, not your Fitbit, to guide your steps each day.** Don't leave him out of your goals—remember, our spiritual, mental, and physical health are intricately connected. He longs to help you feel free in your body so that you can be undistracted in your pursuit and service of him.

Work It Out

Read Isaiah 43:19. Write a letter to the Lord with all he's shown you and keep it someplace where you can reference it when you hit the valley in a few weeks, months, or days even!

What are some ways God can redeem (and use) this part of your story for the benefit of his kingdom, for his glory, and for your good?

Certificate of Commitment

I, _____, am ready to embark on a new journey toward healing my body image. I long to see my body in a different way and to believe that God has called my body good and designed it for a purpose.

Today, I commit to give myself grace as I continue on this journey to freedom. I acknowledge some days will be harder than others. On those days, I will extend kindness and compassion to myself as I learn to believe, think, and treat my body differently. Though the climb may feel long, I will not give up. Neither will I rush my progress or believe the enemy's condemnation when I hear that change isn't happening fast enough.

My desire is to surrender all of my body-focused ideals, hopes, dreams, and plans to Jesus, my Savior. I will endeavor to trust his plans for my life—including his plans for my body and my physical appearance. I lay down every burden I was never meant to carry—including the burden of meeting my own or our culture's standard of beauty.

Thank you, Jesus, for helping me keep this commitment to myself and to you.

Signed: _____

Date: _____

Need More Help?

Think you may be struggling with an eating disorder? Do you have an unhealthy relationship with food or patterns of relating to food that feel difficult to change? It's worth it to get help.

The best counselor is one who you've been referred to by someone you trust. Ask your pastor, women's group leader, or friends for counseling recommendations too.

If that's not an option or the help you need is not nearby, my *Compared to Who?* website keeps a list of licensed eating disorder specialists and non-diet dietitians, many of whom are able to see clients virtually. Visit this page for recommendations: www.improvebodyimage.com/eating-disorder-resources/

Do you feel like you need more support on your body image freedom journey?

Visit improvebodyimage.com for coaching and other opportunities and resources to help and encourage you.

Acknowledgments

Special thanks to the following eating disorder professionals for their input and guidance in the creation of this book: Amy Carlson, MS, RD, LD; Char-Lee Cassel, MS, RDN, ACSM-CEP; Tracy Brown, RD; and Brittany Braswell, MS, RDN, LD.

Thanks also to Erin Todd, Tara Rothwell, Erin Kerry, Shannan Vester, Kassandra Baker, Lauren Platt, Jessica Shreve, Mary DeMuth, Cynthia Ruchti, Jennifer Dukes Lee, Elisa Haugen, Amanda Clawson, and the team at Bethany House for their encouragement and contributions that made this book possible.

· · · ·

As I process the reality of sharing more of my body image story, I'm humbled by God's goodness in using my mess to offer hope to others. Thank you, Jesus, for the journey you've taken me on away from the bondage of serving my image and into the freedom to walk closer with you.

To my husband, Eric, thank you for your stalwart support of my writing career and your encouragement a decade ago to start writing about my body image struggles, even though that was the one topic I wanted to keep a secret. I love you.

Finally, to Zach, Katie, Trevor, and Drew. Though Mom hasn't always done the best job of blending homeschooling with book writing, I praise God that he's allowed me the privilege to be your mother. I love each of you and enjoy seeing the unique ways God has created and gifted you. I pray that you will always find your worth and identity in Christ and be equipped with God's truth so that you may fight the temptation to serve the image idol.

Heather Creekmore writes and speaks hope to thousands of women each week, inspiring them to stop comparing and start living. Heather's *Compared to Who?* podcast is aimed specifically at helping Christian women overcome body image and comparison issues. Her first book, also titled *Compared to Who?*, encourages women to uncover the spiritual root of body image issues and find freedom. Her second release, *The Burden of Better*, offers women a journey into the depths of God's grace to find a way off the treadmill of constant comparison. Heather has been featured on *Fox News, Huff Post, Morning Dose, Church Leaders*, and *For Every Mom*, along with dozens of other shows and podcasts. But she's best recognized from her appearance as a contestant on the Netflix hit show *Nailed It!* Heather and her fighter-pilot-turned-pastor husband, Eric, have four children and live in Austin, Texas.

Connect with Heather at improvebodyimage.com, or listen to the *Compared to Who?* podcast on any podcast app or player.